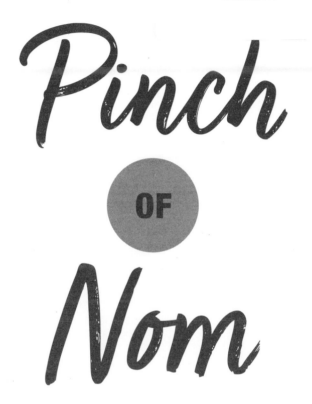

Pinch

OF

Nom

FOOD PLANNER
EVERYDAY LIGHT

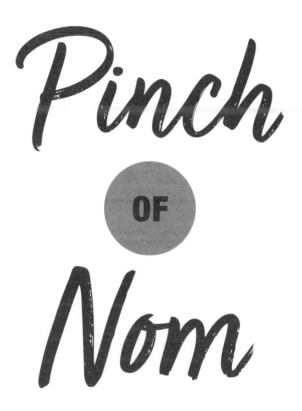

Pinch OF Nom

FOOD PLANNER
EVERYDAY LIGHT

Includes 26 Recipes

bluebird
books for life

First published 2020 by Bluebird
an imprint of Pan Macmillan
The Smithson, 6 Briset Street, London EC1M 5NR

Associated companies throughout the world
www.panmacmillan.com

ISBN   978-1-5290-2644-3

1 3 5 7 9 8 6 4 2

A CIP catalogue record for this book is available from the British Library.

Printed and bound in China.

Publisher Carole Tonkinson
Managing Editor Martha Burley
Senior Production Controller Sarah Badhan
Art Direction, Design and Illustration Emma Wells, Nic&Lou Design
Additional illustrations Shutterstock

Visit www.panmacmillan.com to read more about all our books
and to buy them. You will also find features, author interviews and
news of any author events, and you can sign up for e-newsletters
so that you're always first to hear about our new releases.

CONTENTS

Use this page to scribble down page numbers from the planner – so you can easily refer to a particular week or day of progress, or a recipe you love.

WELCOME TO THE

Pinch OF Nom

FOOD PLANNER

Everyday Light

When starting out on any healthy eating plan, the very best way to keep track of success is to record everything you're eating. Using this one handy planner, you can refer to your complete food intake on a daily basis, while also looking back on previous days and weeks to highlight your best meal choices. We've tried to make this planner as accessible as possible, meaning you can use it whether you're simply calorie counting or following one of the UK's most popular diet plans. This planner should be the perfect tool for keeping track, regardless of the diet plan you are following.

We've made this a 3-month planner as we've added new features and we didn't want to make the planner bigger and bulkier – meaning it's still the perfect size for carrying with you. We know from experience how useful it is to be able to take your planner around with you, so you can record your meals and values as you go. We've included the same number of brilliant recipes though (this time all under 400 calories) to keep you on track as much as possible.

ABOUT
Pinch OF *Nom*

Pinch of Nom started out as a small idea, by Kate and Kay, to share their slimming recipes with friends and family. While the recipes are still at the heart of everything Pinch of Nom does, the community that has grown out of initially just sharing recipes with a select few people has been an amazing and unexpected bonus. It's the community that we listen to and they asked for a planner – we provided! Then we had amazing feedback from our community about the first planner and wanted to make this follow-up as fabulous as possible (with added recipes to boot).

Updated
FEATURES

We're so excited about this new and improved version. Not only can you record your meals for the day, but you can now also plan out your full week of meals and create shopping lists based on your weekly plans. We've included some cute stickers so you can personalize your planners.

And the big news in this planner ... We've also included two *brand-new* recipes a week, created just for you. Although we've packed in more useful content, we didn't want to reduce any of the recipes to make way for it. Because you now have two brand-new recipes a week, you can pop them straight into your meal planner – ready to make in the coming week!

How to
USE THE PLANNER

This book is a beautiful, portable journal for jotting down all of the helpful things for any weight-loss journey. We've given you options to enter your weight at the start of each week, as well as space to jot down your thoughts, goals or aims, plus anything you did well the previous week; anything you want to improve on. We really advise that you take a little time out each week to complete these sections. Not only is it a good way to focus on planning for your upcoming week, but it also gives you a chance to reflect on both the negatives and, more importantly, the positives from the week gone by. This will stand you in good stead going forwards so you're not repeating mistakes, but you're also continuing to do things that have had a positive impact on your weight loss. Although it sounds like a simple step, this mindful approach to your weeks will make a big difference if you use the sections as suggested.

You can also start this planner by jotting down your main aims, plans and goals for the next 3 months. This is your planner; it needs to work for you and inspire you as much as it helps keep track of your food choices. While that may seem like a big ask, just recording your initial hopes for the next 3 months will give you something to reflect on daily to remind yourself of where you want to be. Seeing your own writing stating your aspirations for both yourself and this planner can have a great impact on your motivation to succeed.

It is so important to us that this planner is useful and helps you achieve your goals. In the UK, NHS experts advise that we should be drinking around 1.2 litres of water, which equates to around 8 glasses per day. So we've given you 8 water drops to fill up each time you have a glass of water. This simple marking tool is a great way to keep on plan with your water consumption – something that studies have found can directly help with weight loss. Thirst can often be mistaken for hunger and studies have found that the body's metabolism works at a higher rate when fully hydrated. All great reasons to make a note of how much you are drinking a day. Not to mention being able to congratulate yourself when all 8 drops are filled!

The RECIPES

Compatible with the UK's major diet plans, all of the recipes in the book are calorie-friendly without compromising on taste.

At the heart of everything we do, the recipes are by far the most important and precious to us. Each recipe in this planner has been created to give you recipe ideas that can be used again and again throughout the month.

The recipes have once again been taste tested by our wonderful group of taste testers who were hand-picked from our very own Facebook Group. We wanted to be completely sure that each recipe works and tastes just as good to you as it did when we created it. We also wanted to be sure that the recipes work in unison with people following particular weight-loss plans, as well as calorie counting. We're really proud of the recipes in this planner and we hope you find them useful as part of your cooking and meal-planning routine.

All of the recipes in this book are **Everyday Light**, to accompany our Everyday Light cookbook. But what does Everyday Light mean? Well, the simple answer is that all of the meals in this planner come under 400 calories. But we've made sure to use the right ingredients, so you're still getting a decent portion of food! We didn't want recipes where you only got a teaspoon of food – we wanted the same hearty Pinch of Nom recipes you've come to know and love. If you're following the major diet plans in the UK, all of the recipes can be enjoyed without counting any values, aside from any fibre and dairy allowances.

The majority of these recipes are packed with vegetables and protein – perfect for keeping meals lean, while making sure you're full until your next meal. Of course, for a few extra calories, we have some sides and snacks – but, if you're calorie counting, keep an eye on your main meal calories before adding on the sides.

Freezing Guidelines

Many of our recipes are suitable for freezing (marked with an F, see icons list). When freezing recipes, make sure you freeze as soon as the recipe is cold enough. Use airtight containers or freezer bags that are suitable for the freezer and label them clearly with the recipe name and date. Invest in decent, freezer- and microwave-proof storage containers that seal properly to avoid 'freezer burn'.

Always make sure food is defrosted thoroughly before reheating it, and only reheat food once.

When food has defrosted completely, it should be reheated and eaten within 24 hours. Make sure it is piping hot all the way through. Stir during reheating to ensure this.

Calories and Values

Our calorie counts are all worked out per individual serving. Our meals are calculated with accompaniments in mind, so all the recipes in the planner come in at 400 calories or less *including* accompaniments, so you get a full meal for your 400 cals!

We have not included 'values' from mainstream diet programmes as these are ever-changing and we want this book to be a resource that is always up to date.

Each recipe also displays a set of easily-identifiable icons; explained below.

Our Recipe Icons

V Suitable for vegetarians

F Suitable for freezing. (For all freezer-friendly recipes, we recommend defrosting completely before heating until piping hot.)

GF Suitable for those following a gluten-free diet

3-MONTH
Goals

NAME	STARTING WEIGHT	GOAL WEIGHT

3-MONTH GOAL WEIGHT
We recommend setting an interim goal weight every 3 months to keep motivated and be able to celebrate the smaller goals

REASONS I WANT TO MAKE CHANGES

STATEMENT TO KEEP ME MOTIVATED

One

CHANGE +/-

CURRENT WEIGHT

THIS WEEK I WOULD LIKE TO ACHIEVE

LAST WEEK, THESE THINGS WENT WELL...

REMINDERS FOR THIS WEEK

◯ PLANNED MEALS

◯ SHOPPING DONE

◯ PLANNED EXERCISE

BREAKFAST BOWL

🕐 **5 MINS** | 🍲 **NO-COOK** | ✗ **SERVES 1**

This Breakfast Bowl is a tasty, tropical way to start the day! A twist on the popular smoothie bowl, this version cuts down on the sugars of blended fruit and instead uses a base of protein-filled yoghurt with plenty of high-fibre whole fruits and cereal. It's a lower-calorie, lower-sugar option that still gives you an Instagram-ready breakfast. Perfect!

leave out the cereal

PER SERVING
203 KCAL
19G CARBS

200g fat-free Greek-style yoghurt
1 passion fruit, halved and fruit scooped out
1 tsp granulated sweetener, or to taste
a drop of coconut flavouring
2 chunks of fresh pineapple, thinly sliced
1 fresh strawberry, hulled and thinly sliced
10g high-fibre cereal
1 tsp flaked almonds

Combine the yoghurt, passion fruit, sweetener and coconut flavouring in a bowl.

Arrange the slices of pineapple and strawberry on top, around the outside of the bowl.

Sprinkle the cereal and flaked almonds on top of the yoghurt and serve.

Tip
USE FROZEN FRUIT INSTEAD OF FRESH, IF YOU PREFER. SIMPLY DEFROST AND USE IN THE SAME WAY.

Weekly Meal Planner

	BREAKFAST	LUNCH
MONDAY		
TUESDAY		
WEDNESDAY		
THURSDAY		
FRIDAY		
SATURDAY		
SUNDAY		

Weekly Meal Planner

DINNER	SNACK	NOTES

Day One

BREAKFAST	VALUES
TOTAL	

LUNCH	VALUES
TOTAL	

DINNER	VALUES
TOTAL	

SNACKS AND TREATS	VALUES
TOTAL	

Notes

WATER

Day Two

BREAKFAST	VALUES
TOTAL	

LUNCH	VALUES
TOTAL	

DINNER	VALUES
TOTAL	

SNACKS AND TREATS	VALUES
TOTAL	

'The **Burger in a Bowl** recipe is really easy to follow and very tasty!' SIMONE

WATER

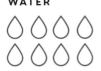

BURGER *in a* BOWL

⏱ **10 MINS** | 🍲 **10 MINS** | ✕ **SERVES 4**

There's no need to run to your calorific local fast-food chain if you fancy a juicy burger. Our Burger in a Bowl has all the flavours and extras you'd expect, but without the high calories. It also has the added bonus of being much easier to eat! Make it your own and add extra pickles or salad vegetables, and enjoy a guilt-free burger experience.

PER SERVING
287 KCAL
7.6G CARBS

low-calorie cooking spray
500g lean minced beef
2 tsp onion granules
½ tsp garlic granules
sea salt and freshly ground
  black pepper
200g fat-free Greek-style
  yoghurt
2 gherkins, 1 finely diced,
  1 sliced, plus extra
  to serve
30g onion, finely chopped
1 tsp English mustard
  powder
2 tsp pickling liquid (from
  a jar of gherkins)
1 tsp tomato puree
100g cherry tomatoes,
  halved
300g little gem lettuce, sliced
30g red onion, finely sliced
80g reduced-fat Cheddar,
  grated

Spray a large frying pan with low-calorie cooking spray and place over a medium heat. Add the mince and fry for 5–6 minutes, until browned, breaking up the meat with a wooden spoon.

Add half the onion granules and all the garlic granules. Season with salt and pepper.

Put the yoghurt, finely diced gherkin, chopped onion, mustard powder, remaining onion granules, pickling liquid and tomato puree in a bowl and mix until combined. Season to taste with salt and pepper.

Arrange the tomatoes and lettuce in a bowl, scatter with the finely sliced red onion, and add the sliced gherkin and grated cheese. Add the browned mince and top with some of the sauce. Serve the rest of the sauce alongside, with extra gherkin.

Day Three

BREAKFAST	VALUES
TOTAL	

LUNCH	VALUES
TOTAL	

DINNER	VALUES
TOTAL	

SNACKS AND TREATS	VALUES
TOTAL	

Notes

WATER

◇ ◇ ◇ ◇
◇ ◇ ◇ ◇

Day Four

Tip
Make planning easier by having your kitchen essentials handy.

BREAKFAST	VALUES
TOTAL	

LUNCH	VALUES
TOTAL	

DINNER	VALUES
TOTAL	

SNACKS AND TREATS	VALUES
TOTAL	

Notes

WATER

◊ ◊ ◊ ◊
◊ ◊ ◊ ◊

Day Five

BREAKFAST	VALUES
TOTAL	

LUNCH	VALUES
TOTAL	

DINNER	VALUES
TOTAL	

SNACKS AND TREATS	VALUES
TOTAL	

Notes

WATER

Day Six

BREAKFAST	VALUES
TOTAL	

LUNCH	VALUES
TOTAL	

DINNER	VALUES
TOTAL	

SNACKS AND TREATS	VALUES
TOTAL	

'A **Breakfast Bowl** is a
tropical dose of yumminess.'
ANNE-MARIE

WATER

WEEK 1

Day Seven

Week
ONE
done!

BREAKFAST	VALUES
TOTAL	

LUNCH	VALUES
TOTAL	

DINNER	VALUES
TOTAL	

SNACKS AND TREATS	VALUES
TOTAL	

Notes

WATER

△ △ △ △
△ △ △ △

SOMETIMES
the
JOURNEY
is as
IMPORTANT
AS THE OUTCOME

Shopping List ❶

....
....
....
....
....
....
....
....
....
....
....
....
....
....
....
....
....
....
....

Shopping List ❷

....
....
....
....
....
....
....
....
....
....
....
....
....
....
....
....
....
....
....

Shopping List ②

....
....
....
....
....
....
....
....
....
....
....
....
....
....
....
....
....
....

Shopping List ①

....
....
....
....
....
....
....
....
....
....
....
....
....
....
....
....
....

It's

Never
TOO
LATE TO

CHANGE OLD

Habits

WEEK
Two

CHANGE +/-

CURRENT WEIGHT

THIS WEEK I WOULD LIKE TO ACHIEVE

LAST WEEK, THESE THINGS WENT WELL...

REMINDERS FOR THIS WEEK

○ **PLANNED MEALS**

○ **SHOPPING DONE**

○ **PLANNED EXERCISE**

PHILLY CHEESESTEAK PASTA

⏱ **5 MINS** | 🍲 **17 MINS** | ✕ **SERVES 4**

Philly Cheesesteak is, as you'd expect from the name, a Philadelphia staple. We are absolutely down with the flavour combination of cheese and steak, so we took out the sandwich and added the flavours to pasta for a filling, delicious meal. Using minced beef instead of steak makes it lower in calories and cost!

PER SERVING
397 KCAL
51.6G CARBS

200g dried pasta
low-calorie cooking spray
2 onions, peeled and finely chopped
2 peppers, deseeded and sliced into thin strips
200g 5%-fat beef mince
2 tsp Worcestershire sauce
2 tsp garlic granules
300g mushrooms, thinly sliced
sea salt and freshly ground black pepper
150ml beef stock (1 beef stock cube dissolved in 150ml boiling water)
150g light spreadable cheese
40g reduced-fat Cheddar

Cook the pasta in a saucepan according to the packet instructions.

While the pasta is cooking, spray a frying pan with low-calorie cooking spray. Cook the onions and peppers over a medium heat for 5 minutes, until the onions have softened. Add the beef mince, Worcestershire sauce and garlic and cook for a further 3 minutes, until the beef has browned. Add the mushrooms to the frying pan and cook for another 3 minutes. Season to taste with salt and pepper.

Drain the pasta and pour in the beef mix. Mix in the beef stock and the spreadable cheese. If your frying pan isn't ovenproof, transfer the mix into a roasting dish and grate the Cheddar on top. Place in the middle of the oven for 5 minutes, until the cheese has melted, then take out and serve. (You can also cool and freeze for another day.)

Tip
LIGHTEN UP THIS DISH FURTHER BY LEAVING OUT THE CHEESE ON TOP; JUST SERVE AFTER MIXING IN THE SPREADABLE CHEESE AND STOCK.

Weekly Meal Planner

	BREAKFAST	LUNCH
MONDAY		
TUESDAY		
WEDNESDAY		
THURSDAY		
FRIDAY		
SATURDAY		
SUNDAY		

Weekly Meal Planner

DINNER	SNACK	NOTES

Day One

BREAKFAST	VALUES
TOTAL	

LUNCH	VALUES
TOTAL	

DINNER	VALUES
TOTAL	

SNACKS AND TREATS	VALUES
TOTAL	

Notes

WATER

Day Two

BREAKFAST	VALUES
TOTAL	

LUNCH	VALUES
TOTAL	

DINNER	VALUES
TOTAL	

SNACKS AND TREATS	VALUES
TOTAL	

Notes

WATER

△ △ △ △
△ △ △ △

SALMON FATTOUSH

🕐 15 MINS | 🍲 15 MINS | ✗ SERVES 4

In this twist on a classic Middle Eastern salad, we have combined the citrus flavours of sumac with fresh mint and parsley to create a salad packed full of flavour and a vibrant mix of healthy ingredients. Baked pitta 'croutons' add crunch and filling power, making this perfect for a packed lunch on a workday.

PER SERVING
339 KCAL
28G CARBS

low-calorie cooking spray
2 medium salmon fillets (about 150g each), skin removed
1 tsp sumac
2 wholemeal pitta breads
1 cucumber
300g cherry tomatoes
150g radishes
½ medium red onion
100g fat-free natural yoghurt
10g fresh mint leaves, finely chopped
10g fresh flat-leaf parsley, finely chopped
½ tsp garlic granules
juice of ½ lemon
¼ tsp granulated sweetener or sugar (optional)
sea salt and freshly ground black pepper
2 little gem lettuces, washed, shaken dry and torn into chunks

Preheat the oven to 180°C (fan 160°C/gas mark 4) and lightly spray a baking tray with low-calorie cooking spray.

Dust the salmon fillets with half of the sumac and place on the baking tray.

Spray the pitta breads with low-calorie cooking spray and place them on the baking tray with the salmon. Place the salmon and breads in the oven and bake for 15 minutes.

Meanwhile, prepare the salad.

Cut the cucumber in half lengthways, scoop out the seeds with a teaspoon and discard, and cut the cucumber into half-moon-shaped slices. Halve the tomatoes, quarter each radish and roughly chop the red onion.

Now, make the dressing. Mix the yoghurt, mint, parsley, garlic granules, lemon juice and sweetener (if using) in a bowl or small jug. Add 2–3 tablespoons of water to thin the yoghurt to a salad dressing consistency and season with a pinch of salt and some black pepper.

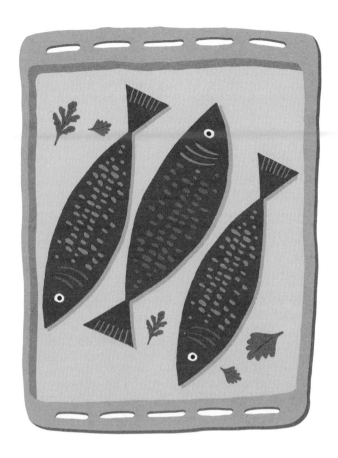

Arrange the salad ingredients in four bowls with the chunks of lettuce.

Tip
SUBSTITUTE THE SALMON FOR A SMALL SKINLESS CHICKEN BREAST, IF YOU PREFER, CHECKING IT IS COOKED THROUGH BEFORE REMOVING IT FROM THE OVEN.

When the salmon is cooked, remove the tray from the oven and flake the salmon equally among the four salad bowls.

Break the baked pitta into small pieces – it should be crisp – and use it to top each salad. Drizzle over most of the dressing (serving the rest alongside), sprinkle the remaining sumac over the salads and serve.

Day Three

BREAKFAST	VALUES
TOTAL	

LUNCH	VALUES
TOTAL	

DINNER	VALUES
TOTAL	

SNACKS AND TREATS	VALUES
TOTAL	

*'Delicious. Had the **Salmon Fattoush** for lunch and dinner.'*
JANET

WATER

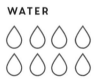

Day Four

BREAKFAST	VALUES
TOTAL	

LUNCH	VALUES
TOTAL	

DINNER	VALUES
TOTAL	

SNACKS AND TREATS	VALUES
TOTAL	

Notes

WATER

Day Five

BREAKFAST	VALUES
TOTAL	

LUNCH	VALUES
TOTAL	

DINNER	VALUES
TOTAL	

SNACKS AND TREATS	VALUES
TOTAL	

Notes

_____

_____

_____

WATER

○ ○ ○ ○

○ ○ ○ ○

Day Six

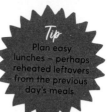

Tip
Plan easy lunches – perhaps reheated leftovers from the previous day's meals.

BREAKFAST	VALUES
TOTAL	

LUNCH	VALUES
TOTAL	

DINNER	VALUES
TOTAL	

SNACKS AND TREATS	VALUES
TOTAL	

Notes

WATER

◊ ◊ ◊ ◊
◊ ◊ ◊ ◊

Day Seven

BREAKFAST	VALUES
TOTAL	

LUNCH	VALUES
TOTAL	

DINNER	VALUES
TOTAL	

SNACKS AND TREATS	VALUES
TOTAL	

'Absolutely loved the **Salmon Fattoush**.
So fresh and tasty, easy to prepare and
the dressing is divine!' **SHIRLEY**

WATER

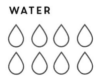

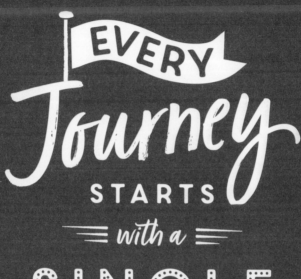

EVERY *Journey* STARTS ~ *with a* ~ SINGLE STEP

Three

CHANGE +/-

CURRENT WEIGHT

THIS WEEK I WOULD LIKE TO ACHIEVE

LAST WEEK, THESE THINGS WENT WELL...

REMINDERS FOR THIS WEEK

◯ PLANNED MEALS

◯ SHOPPING DONE

◯ PLANNED EXERCISE

FISH CURRY

🕐 **10 MINS** | 🍲 **15 MINS** | ✕ **SERVES 4**

If it swims, it slims! Making a simple swap from meat to fish in a curry means you shave off calories while having the added benefit of fish being so tasty. This simple fish curry uses just a few ingredients to make a super-quick and hearty meal. You can use any firm white fish and change the spice level by adding more or less curry powder to suit your taste.

PER SERVING
143 KCAL
4G CARBS

low-calorie cooking spray
60g onion, sliced
2 garlic cloves, crushed
1 tbsp curry powder
1 tsp ground turmeric
1 tbsp tomato puree
600g skinless, boneless
    cod loin, cut into 2cm
    (¾ in) cubes
2 tsp lemon juice
400ml water
4 tbsp chopped fresh
    coriander
sea salt and freshly ground
    black pepper

TO ACCOMPANY
(optional)

125g cooked rice per
    portion (+ 173 kcal
    per serving)

Spray a deep frying pan with some low-calorie cooking spray, place over a medium heat. Add the onions and garlic and cook for about 5 minutes until softened.

Add the curry powder and turmeric to the pan and cook for 1 minute, then add all the remaining ingredients, saving a little coriander for a garnish when cooked.

Bring to the boil, stirring very gently so as not to break up the fish, then turn down the heat to low and cook gently for 8–9 minutes, until the fish is opaque and flakes apart. Season to taste and remove from the heat.

Scatter with the reserved coriander and serve with rice or your choice of accompaniment.

Weekly Meal Planner

	BREAKFAST	LUNCH
MONDAY		
TUESDAY		
WEDNESDAY		
THURSDAY		
FRIDAY		
SATURDAY		
SUNDAY		

Weekly Meal Planner

DINNER	SNACK	NOTES

Day One

BREAKFAST	VALUES
TOTAL	

LUNCH	VALUES
TOTAL	

DINNER	VALUES
TOTAL	

SNACKS AND TREATS	VALUES
TOTAL	

Notes

WATER

Day Two

BREAKFAST	VALUES
TOTAL	

LUNCH	VALUES
TOTAL	

DINNER	VALUES
TOTAL	

SNACKS AND TREATS	VALUES
TOTAL	

'The **Fish Curry** is such a quick,
easy-to-follow, nutritious dish.'
SHIRLEY

WATER

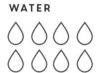

Day Three

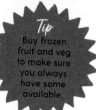

BREAKFAST	VALUES
TOTAL	

LUNCH	VALUES
TOTAL	

DINNER	VALUES
TOTAL	

SNACKS AND TREATS	VALUES
TOTAL	

Notes

WATER

Day Four

BREAKFAST	VALUES
TOTAL	

LUNCH	VALUES
TOTAL	

DINNER	VALUES
TOTAL	

SNACKS AND TREATS	VALUES
TOTAL	

Notes

WATER

Day Five

BREAKFAST	VALUES
TOTAL	

LUNCH	VALUES
TOTAL	

DINNER	VALUES
TOTAL	

SNACKS AND TREATS	VALUES
TOTAL	

'The **Lemon Drizzle Oat Muffins**
*are really nice – felt like having
a treat.'* **AMY**

WATER

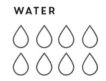

Day Six

BREAKFAST	VALUES
TOTAL	

LUNCH	VALUES
TOTAL	

DINNER	VALUES
TOTAL	

SNACKS AND TREATS	VALUES
TOTAL	

Notes

WATER

◇ ◇ ◇ ◇
◇ ◇ ◇ ◇

LEMON DRIZZLE OAT MUFFINS

🕐 **15 MINS** | 🍲 **15 MINS** | ✗ **MAKES 12**

These tasty muffins are the perfect sweet fix, whether you're looking for a between-meals snack, a dessert, or want to serve them as part of an afternoon tea. Using oats instead of flour makes a filling but low-calorie cake while not compromising on the delicious lemon-drizzly flavour.

PER MUFFIN
60 KCAL
4G CARBS

Equipment
12-hole muffin tin

50g granulated sweetener
3 medium eggs
2 tsp lemon extract
80g Ready Brek
grated or finely sliced zest
    and juice of 2 lemons

Preheat the oven to 170°C (fan 150°C/gas mark 3) and line a 12-hole muffin tin with twelve cases.

Put most of the sweetener into a large mixing bowl (keep back 1 teaspoon for the drizzle) and add the eggs and the lemon extract. Whisk with an electric hand whisk for 7–8 minutes until very pale yellow and thick – the mixture should leave a ribbon trail in the bowl when you lift the whisk up.

Using a spatula, carefully fold in the Ready Brek and half the lemon zest. Try not to over-mix: you don't want to knock all the air out of the mixture.

Gently divide the mixture among the muffin cases and bake in the oven for 15 minutes until golden.

Meanwhile, put the lemon juice in a small saucepan with most of the remaining lemon zest and the remaining teaspoon of sweetener.

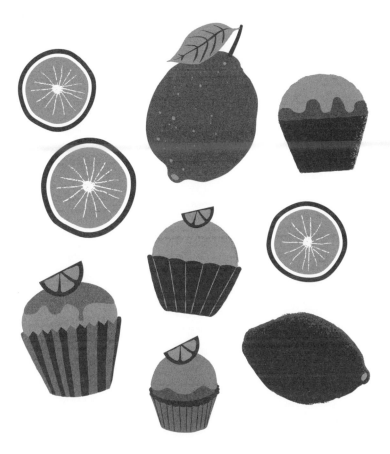

Heat until the drizzle starts to boil and the sweetener has dissolved, then remove from the heat.

Test if the muffins are cooked: a skewer inserted into the middle of a muffin should come out clean. Remove from the oven, place the muffins onto a wire rack and poke a few holes with a skewer into the top of each. Pour the lemon drizzle evenly over each muffin, top with a little leftover zest, and leave to cool before serving.

The muffins can be frozen once cooled.

Tips

• BLITZ UP SOME PORRIDGE OATS UNTIL VERY FINE INSTEAD OF USING READY BREK.

• BE SURE TO USE A GRANULATED SWEETENER THAT HAS A LIKE-FOR-LIKE WEIGHT WITH SUGAR.

Day Seven

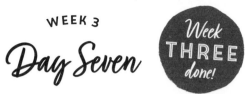

Week THREE done!

BREAKFAST	VALUES
TOTAL	

LUNCH	VALUES
TOTAL	

DINNER	VALUES
TOTAL	

SNACKS AND TREATS	VALUES
TOTAL	

Notes

_____

_____

_____

WATER

○ ○ ○ ○
○ ○ ○ ○

Shopping List 1

....
....
....
....
....
....
....
....
....
....
....
....
....
....
....
....
....
....

Shopping List 2

....
....
....
....
....
....
....
....
....
....
....
....
....
....
....
....
....
....

Shopping List 2

....
....
....
....
....
....
....
....
....
....
....
....
....
....
....
....
....
....
....

Shopping List 1

....
....
....
....
....
....
....
....
....
....
....
....
....
....
....
....
....
....
....

. YOU'VE .

GOT

this

WEEK

Four

CHANGE +/-

CURRENT WEIGHT

THIS WEEK I WOULD LIKE TO ACHIEVE

LAST WEEK, THESE THINGS WENT WELL...

REMINDERS FOR THIS WEEK

◯ PLANNED MEALS

◯ SHOPPING DONE

◯ PLANNED EXERCISE

CHILLI BEEF SOFT TACOS

🕐 **10 MINS** | 🍲 **20 MINS** | ✗ **SERVES 4**

Our version of this Mexican classic uses the soft leaves from a little gem lettuce to create the taco shell, and combines cooling yoghurt with a spicy jalapeño kick. They are really easy to adapt to your taste – make them as fiery or as mild as you like!

GF 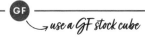 use a GF stock cube

PER SERVING
323 KCAL
25G CARBS

low-calorie cooking spray
250g lean minced beef
60g onion, finely diced
1 red pepper, deseeded
   and finely diced
260g drained tinned
   sweetcorn
205g tin kidney beans in
   chilli sauce
2 garlic cloves, crushed
1 tsp dried chilli flakes
2 tsp ground cumin
1 tsp smoked paprika
2 tbsp tomato puree
1 beef stock cube
sea salt and freshly ground
   black pepper
300g little gem lettuce
100g fat-free Greek-style
   yoghurt
80g reduced-fat Cheddar,
   grated
50g sliced jalapeños in
   brine, drained

Spray a large frying pan with low-calorie cooking spray and place over a medium heat. Add the minced beef, onion and diced pepper and fry for 7–8 minutes until the beef starts to brown, breaking up the mince with a wooden spoon.

Add the sweetcorn, kidney beans in chilli sauce, garlic, chilli flakes, ground cumin, paprika and tomato puree, crumble in the stock cube and mix well. Season with salt and pepper and simmer over a low heat for 10–12 minutes until the sauce is rich and the meat is tender.

Separate the gem lettuce into leaves and arrange on a plate and spoon some of the beef chilli mixture into each leaf. Top each filled lettuce 'taco' with some Greek yoghurt, grated cheese and jalapeños.

Tips

• SCATTER WITH SLICED RED CHILLI, IF YOU LIKE.

• YOU COULD SERVE THESE IN SOFT TACO SHELLS INSTEAD – JUST CHECK THE NUTRITIONAL VALUES.

Weekly Meal Planner

	BREAKFAST	LUNCH
MONDAY		
TUESDAY		
WEDNESDAY		
THURSDAY		
FRIDAY		
SATURDAY		
SUNDAY		

Weekly Meal Planner

DINNER	SNACK	NOTES

Day One

BREAKFAST	VALUES
TOTAL	

LUNCH	VALUES
TOTAL	

DINNER	VALUES
TOTAL	

SNACKS AND TREATS	VALUES
TOTAL	

Notes

WATER

WEEK 4

Day Two

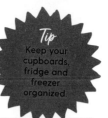

Tip
Keep your cupboards, fridge and freezer organized.

BREAKFAST	**VALUES**
TOTAL	

LUNCH	**VALUES**
TOTAL	

DINNER	**VALUES**
TOTAL	

SNACKS AND TREATS	**VALUES**
TOTAL	

Notes

WATER

◇ ◇ ◇ ◇
◇ ◇ ◇ ◇

Day Three

BREAKFAST	VALUES
TOTAL	

LUNCH	VALUES
TOTAL	

DINNER	VALUES
TOTAL	

SNACKS AND TREATS	VALUES
TOTAL	

'Absolutely loved the
Chilli Beef Soft Tacos!'
SALLY

WATER

Day Four

BREAKFAST	VALUES
TOTAL	

LUNCH	VALUES
TOTAL	

DINNER	VALUES
TOTAL	

SNACKS AND TREATS	VALUES
TOTAL	

Notes

WATER

◇ ◇ ◇ ◇
◇ ◇ ◇ ◇

ITALIAN WHITE BEAN SOUP

🕐 **15 MINS** | 🍲 **30 MINS** | ✕ **SERVES 4**

Packed with vegetables, beans and tasty herbs, this hearty soup brings a taste of Italy to lunchtime. It's perfect for a cold winter's day, to help make you feel you're escaping the chill! Add a bread roll for a more substantial meal.

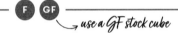 F GF → use a GF stock cube

PER SERVING
209 KCAL
23G CARBS

low-calorie cooking spray
4 bacon medallions, cut into 1cm (½ in) pieces
1 onion, diced
1 large carrot, diced
1 celery stick, diced
4 garlic cloves, minced
10g fresh thyme, leaves chopped
1 litre chicken stock (2 chicken stock cubes dissolved in 1 litre boiling water)
1 bay leaf
2 x 400g tins cannellini beans, drained and rinsed
75g kale, tough stems removed and leaves roughly chopped
juice of ½ lemon
freshly ground black pepper

Spray a saucepan with low-calorie cooking spray and place over a medium heat. Add the bacon, onion, carrot and celery and sauté for 5 minutes, until the onion has softened.

Add the garlic and thyme and cook for another minute.

Pour in the stock, bring to the boil, then reduce the heat, pop in the bay leaf and simmer for 20 minutes.

Check the carrots are cooked, then add the beans and the kale and cook for another 5 minutes.

To thicken the soup, remove the bay leaf, take out a couple of ladles of soup and blitz it in a blender. Return the blitzed soup to the pan and stir well.

Add the lemon juice and a twist of black pepper and serve.

 Tip
YOU COULD LEAVE OUT THE BACON AND CHANGE TO VEG STOCK TO MAKE THIS A VEGGIE SOUP.

Day Five

BREAKFAST	VALUES
TOTAL	

LUNCH	VALUES
TOTAL	

DINNER	VALUES
TOTAL	

SNACKS AND TREATS	VALUES
TOTAL	

Notes

WATER

67

Day Six

BREAKFAST	VALUES
TOTAL	

LUNCH	VALUES
TOTAL	

DINNER	VALUES
TOTAL	

SNACKS AND TREATS	VALUES
TOTAL	

Notes

WATER

Day Seven

BREAKFAST	VALUES
TOTAL	

LUNCH	VALUES
TOTAL	

DINNER	VALUES
TOTAL	

SNACKS AND TREATS	VALUES
TOTAL	

*'The whole family loved the **Italian White Bean Soup** – it made for a perfect autumn warmer with crusty bread after a nice walk with the dog!'* **CAROLINE**

WATER

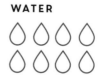

CHANGE +/-

CURRENT WEIGHT

THIS WEEK I WOULD LIKE TO ACHIEVE

LAST WEEK, THESE THINGS WENT WELL...

REMINDERS FOR THIS WEEK

○ PLANNED MEALS

○ SHOPPING DONE

○ PLANNED EXERCISE

BABY ROASTIES

🕐 **1 MIN** | 🍲 **40 MINS** | ✕ **SERVES 4**

This side dish is perfectly for pairing with a mid-week dinner; there's no need for peeling or chopping and it's super-quick and tasty so you don't have to spend an age prepping for your roast potato fix! For far less effort and with no need for all the oil and fat of standard roasties, this side is set to become a firm favourite.

PER SERVING
178 KCAL
37G CARBS

1kg baby potatoes
low-calorie cooking spray
1 tsp dried thyme
½ tsp garlic granules
sea salt and freshly ground black pepper
1 tsp chopped fresh chives, to serve (optional)

Tip
SWAP THE THYME FOR OTHER HERBS AND SPICES, DEPENDING ON THE MEAL YOU ARE HAVING. ROSEMARY, PAPRIKA, CHILLI POWDER ... THE POSSIBILITIES ARE ENDLESS!

Preheat the oven to 220°C (fan 200°C/gas mark 7).

Try to use potatoes that are roughly all the same size. If there are a few that are a lot bigger, cut them in half.

Put the potatoes in a roasting dish and spray well with low-calorie cooking spray. Toss to coat.

Sprinkle over the thyme and garlic and season with salt and pepper. Toss the potatoes so they are evenly coated.

Roast the potatoes in the oven for 40 minutes. When they are cooked the outsides will be golden and crispy and the insides will be soft and tender when pronged with a fork.

Serve with a sprinkle of chopped chives, if you like. These can be frozen once cooled. Defrost thoroughly before reheating.

Weekly Meal Planner

	BREAKFAST	LUNCH
MONDAY		
TUESDAY		
WEDNESDAY		
THURSDAY		
FRIDAY		
SATURDAY		
SUNDAY		

Weekly Meal Planner

DINNER	SNACK	NOTES

Day One

BREAKFAST	VALUES
TOTAL	

LUNCH	VALUES
TOTAL	

DINNER	VALUES
TOTAL	

SNACKS AND TREATS	VALUES
TOTAL	

Notes

WATER

Day Two

BREAKFAST	VALUES
TOTAL	

LUNCH	VALUES
TOTAL	

DINNER	VALUES
TOTAL	

SNACKS AND TREATS	VALUES
TOTAL	

Notes
_____

WATER

◇ ◇ ◇ ◇
◇ ◇ ◇ ◇

Day Three

BREAKFAST	VALUES
TOTAL	

LUNCH	VALUES
TOTAL	

DINNER	VALUES
TOTAL	

SNACKS AND TREATS	VALUES
TOTAL	

Notes

WATER

Day Four

BREAKFAST	VALUES
TOTAL	

LUNCH	VALUES
TOTAL	

DINNER	VALUES
TOTAL	

SNACKS AND TREATS	VALUES
TOTAL	

'The **Baby Roasties** are cracking for turning something ordinary into something amazing. They made my meal more enjoyable.' **CHARLI MARIE**

WATER

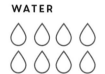

WEEK 5

Day Five

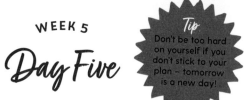

Tip
Don't be too hard on yourself if you don't stick to your plan – tomorrow is a new day!

BREAKFAST	VALUES
TOTAL	

LUNCH	VALUES
TOTAL	

DINNER	VALUES
TOTAL	

SNACKS AND TREATS	VALUES
TOTAL	

Notes

WATER

○ ○ ○ ○
○ ○ ○ ○

Day Six

BREAKFAST	VALUES
TOTAL	

LUNCH	VALUES
TOTAL	

DINNER	VALUES
TOTAL	

SNACKS AND TREATS	VALUES
TOTAL	

Notes

WATER

○ ○ ○ ○
○ ○ ○ ○

MUSHROOM BURGERS

🕐 **15 MINS** | 🍲 **16–18 MINS** | ✕ **SERVES 4**

We all know that a vegetarian version of a meat dish is almost always lower in calories, but it can be hard to get that juicy, meaty flavour with meat-free meals. In these tasty veggie burgers, however, we've used beans for protein and mushrooms for bold flavour, so even the most dedicated carnivore won't miss the meat.

→ use GF rolls and soy sauce

PER SERVING
290 KCAL
37G CARBS

1 small courgette, grated
low-calorie cooking spray
½ red onion, finely chopped
250g mushrooms, finely chopped
1 tsp dried thyme
2 tsp garlic granules
1 tbsp soy sauce
1 x 400g tin black beans, drained and rinsed
1 egg yolk
seat salt and freshly ground black pepper
½ tsp xantham gum (optional)
4 x 60g seeded wholemeal rolls
mixed salad, to serve

Wrap the grated courgette in a clean tea towel and squeeze out any liquid.

Spray a large non-stick frying pan with low-calorie cooking spray, place over a medium heat, add the onion, mushrooms and courgette and sauté for 5–10 minutes, until the liquid that the mushrooms release has evaporated. It is important to have a dry mix so the burgers don't fall apart.

When all the liquid has evaporated, add the thyme, garlic granules and soy sauce and cook for 1 more minute. Remove from the heat and allow to cool.

Meanwhile, dry the beans well with some kitchen towel then put in a bowl and roughly mash with a fork.

Mix the vegetables and beans together with the egg yolk and season well with salt and pepper. Add the xantham gum, if using (this will help hold the burgers together while cooking).

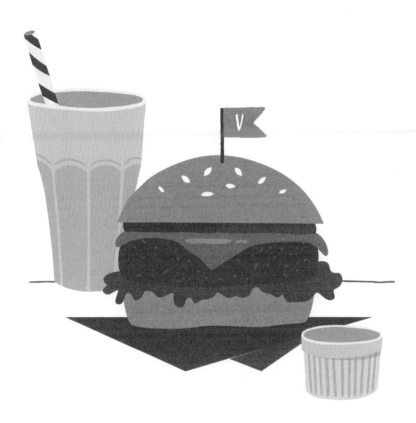

Wipe out the frying pan and give it another spray with low-calorie cooking spray. Place over a medium heat.

Form the burger mix into four patties and carefully place them in the pan. Fry the burgers for 3–4 minutes on each side until browned. Turn them carefully, and only once, to prevent them breaking up.

Serve the burgers in wholemeal rolls, with plenty of mixed salad.

Day Seven

Week **FIVE** done!

BREAKFAST	VALUES
TOTAL	

LUNCH	VALUES
TOTAL	

DINNER	VALUES
TOTAL	

SNACKS AND TREATS	VALUES
TOTAL	

'The **Mushroom Burgers** make a fantastic alternative to beef.'
DEIRDRE

WATER

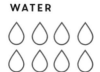

Shopping List 1

....
....
....
....
....
....
....
....
....
....
....
....
....
....
....
....
....
....

Shopping List 2

....
....
....
....
....
....
....
....
....
....
....
....
....
....
....
....
....
....

Shopping List 2

....
....
....
....
....
....
....
....
....
....
....
....
....
....
....
....
....
....
....

Shopping List 1

....
....
....
....
....
....
....
....
....
....
....
....
....
....
....
....
....
....
....

Small
CHANGES
≡ ADD UP TO ≡
BIG
RESULTS

WEEK
Six

CHANGE +/-

CURRENT WEIGHT

THIS WEEK I WOULD LIKE TO ACHIEVE

LAST WEEK, THESE THINGS WENT WELL...

REMINDERS FOR THIS WEEK

◯ PLANNED MEALS

◯ SHOPPING DONE

◯ PLANNED EXERCISE

TUNA PASTA QUICHE

🕐 **15 MINS** | 🍲 **35 MINS** | ✗ **SERVES 6**

Pasta and quiche might not sound like a natural combination, but trust us, it really does work! It makes the quiche taste extra creamy and adds substance that defies the low calorie count. You can eat it warm, straight from the oven, but in our opinion it is even better cold for lunch the next day!

PER SERVING
231 KCAL
14G CARBS

Equipment
26cm (10in) quiche dish

75g macaroni or other
    small pasta shapes
sea salt and freshly ground
    black pepper
low-calorie cooking spray
1 medium red onion, sliced
1 medium red pepper, halved,
    deseeded and chopped
6 large eggs
250g fat-free cottage cheese
1 x 145g tin of tuna in spring
    water, drained
60g reduced-fat mature
    Cheddar, grated
mixed salad, to serve

Cook the macaroni in a saucepan of salted boiling water according to the packet instructions. Preheat the oven to 180°C (fan 160°C/gas mark 4).

While the pasta is cooking, spray a frying pan with low-calorie cooking spray, place over a medium heat and add the onion and pepper. Sauté for 3–4 minutes, until soft.

Crack the eggs into a large bowl and beat thoroughly. If you prefer a smoother texture, blitz the cottage cheese in a blender until smooth. Add to the eggs and beat until well combined.

When the pasta is cooked, drain well, then stir into the egg and cheese mixture, along with the rest of the ingredients.

Spray the quiche dish with low-calorie cooking spray and pour in the mixture. Cook in the oven for 30–35 minutes, until the centre has set.

Remove from the oven and serve warm or cold. This can be frozen once cooled – defrost thoroughly before reheating.

Weekly Meal Planner

	BREAKFAST	LUNCH
MONDAY		
TUESDAY		
WEDNESDAY		
THURSDAY		
FRIDAY		
SATURDAY		
SUNDAY		

Weekly Meal Planner

DINNER	SNACK	NOTES

Day One

BREAKFAST	VALUES
TOTAL	

LUNCH	VALUES
TOTAL	

DINNER	VALUES
TOTAL	

SNACKS AND TREATS	VALUES
TOTAL	

Notes

WATER

○ ○ ○ ○
○ ○ ○ ○

Day Two

BREAKFAST	VALUES
TOTAL	

LUNCH	VALUES
TOTAL	

DINNER	VALUES
TOTAL	

SNACKS AND TREATS	VALUES
TOTAL	

'The **Pork Pizzaiola** is wonderful and absolutely delicious. Easy to make, everyday ingredients, and quick to cook.'
LYN

WATER

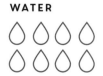

WEEK 6
Day Three

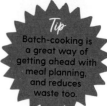

Tip
Batch-cooking is a great way of getting ahead with meal planning, and reduces waste too.

BREAKFAST	VALUES
TOTAL	

LUNCH	VALUES
TOTAL	

DINNER	VALUES
TOTAL	

SNACKS AND TREATS	VALUES
TOTAL	

Notes
_____
_____
_____

WATER
◇ ◇ ◇ ◇
◇ ◇ ◇ ◇

Day Four

BREAKFAST	VALUES
TOTAL	

LUNCH	VALUES
TOTAL	

DINNER	VALUES
TOTAL	

SNACKS AND TREATS	VALUES
TOTAL	

Notes

WATER

○ ○ ○ ○
○ ○ ○ ○

Day Five

BREAKFAST	VALUES
	TOTAL

LUNCH	VALUES
	TOTAL

DINNER	VALUES
	TOTAL

SNACKS AND TREATS	VALUES
	TOTAL

> 'Pork Pizzaiola *made
> a delicious meal.*'
> **SALLY**

WATER

Day Six

BREAKFAST	VALUES
TOTAL	

LUNCH	VALUES
TOTAL	

DINNER	VALUES
TOTAL	

SNACKS AND TREATS	VALUES
TOTAL	

Notes

WATER

◊ ◊ ◊ ◊
◊ ◊ ◊ ◊

PORK PIZZAIOLA

🕐 15 MINS | 🍲 35 MINS | ✕ SERVES 4

So-called because the pork steaks are cooked in a rich, tomatoey 'pizza-style' sauce, making them beautifully tender. With its added veggies, and an accompaniment of fresh, lemony green beans, this pork pizzaiola is a quick and easy, yet super-tasty weeknight meal.

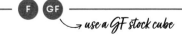 → use a GF stock cube

PER SERVING
278 KCAL
14G CARBS

low-calorie cooking spray
4 lean pork steaks (about 135g each), trimmed of all visible fat
1 medium onion, chopped
1 medium red pepper, halved, deseeded and chopped
1 large carrot, cut into small dice
4 garlic cloves, finely chopped or grated
10g fresh oregano, leaves chopped
1 x 400g tin chopped tomatoes
100ml chicken stock (1 chicken stock cube dissolved in 100ml boiling water)
sea salt and freshly ground black pepper
300g trimmed green beans
½ lemon
15g grated Parmesan

Spray a large lidded heavy-based frying pan with low-calorie cooking spray and place over a high heat. Add the pork steaks and brown them for 2 minutes on each side. Remove the pork from the pan and place to one side.

Reduce the heat to medium. Add the vegetables to the pan and sauté for 3–4 minutes, then add the garlic and cook for 1 minute. Stir in the oregano, tomatoes and stock, bring to the boil, then reduce the heat, cover and simmer for 12 minutes.

Stir a pinch of black pepper into the sauce. Return the pork steaks to the pan with the sauce, cover and cook for 10–15 minutes, until the carrots are soft and the pork is cooked through. (The cooked pork and sauce can be frozen at this point.)

Bring a saucepan of salted water to the boil and cook the green beans for 5 minutes, or until cooked. Drain the beans, squeeze over the lemon juice, and season with a little pepper. Divide the pork and beans among four plates, sprinkle over the Parmesan and serve.

Day Seven

BREAKFAST	VALUES
TOTAL	

LUNCH	VALUES
TOTAL	

DINNER	VALUES
TOTAL	

SNACKS AND TREATS	VALUES
TOTAL	

Notes

WATER

◇ ◇ ◇ ◇
◇ ◇ ◇ ◇

WEEK
Seven

CHANGE +/-

CURRENT WEIGHT

THIS WEEK I WOULD LIKE TO ACHIEVE

LAST WEEK, THESE THINGS WENT WELL...

REMINDERS FOR THIS WEEK

○ PLANNED MEALS

○ SHOPPING DONE

○ PLANNED EXERCISE

REMEMBER WHY · YOU Started

Weekly Meal Planner

	BREAKFAST	LUNCH
MONDAY		
TUESDAY		
WEDNESDAY		
THURSDAY		
FRIDAY		
SATURDAY		
SUNDAY		

Weekly Meal Planner

DINNER	SNACK	NOTES

WEEK 7

Day One

BREAKFAST	VALUES
TOTAL	

LUNCH	VALUES
TOTAL	

DINNER	VALUES
TOTAL	

SNACKS AND TREATS	VALUES
TOTAL	

Notes

WATER

Day Two

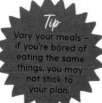

Tip
Vary your meals –
if you're bored of
eating the same
things, you may
not stick to
your plan.

BREAKFAST	VALUES
TOTAL	

LUNCH	VALUES
TOTAL	

DINNER	VALUES
TOTAL	

SNACKS AND TREATS	VALUES
TOTAL	

Notes

WATER

◇ ◇ ◇ ◇
◇ ◇ ◇ ◇

Day Three

BREAKFAST	VALUES
TOTAL	

LUNCH	VALUES
TOTAL	

DINNER	VALUES
TOTAL	

SNACKS AND TREATS	VALUES
TOTAL	

'The **Mojo Beef Skewers** *made a lush addition to a barbecue.*'
ZARA

WATER

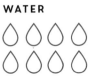

Day Four

BREAKFAST	VALUES
TOTAL	

LUNCH	VALUES
TOTAL	

DINNER	VALUES
TOTAL	

SNACKS AND TREATS	VALUES
TOTAL	

Notes

WATER

MOJO BEEF SKEWERS
with CITRUS RICE

🕐 **15 MINS*** | 🍲 **25 MINS** | ✕ **SERVES 4**
* PLUS MINIMUM 1 HOUR MARINATING

These tender steak chunks marinated in citrus, garlic and a little Cuban-inspired spicing are great for a barbecue or to cook indoors on a griddle pan. You can amend the spicing to your taste – if you like a kick, just add a little more chilli. Serve with the zingy citrus rice.

GF

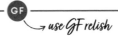 *use GF relish*

PER SERVING
381 KCAL
46G CARBS

Equipment
8 skewers

grated zest and juice of
  1 orange
grated zest and juice of
  1 lime, plus lime wedges
  to serve
2 tsp garlic granules
2 tsp Henderson's relish or
  Worcestershire sauce
1 tsp dried oregano
½ tsp ground cumin
pinch of dried chilli flakes
  (optional)
pinch of granulated
  sweetener or sugar
  (optional)
500g lean quick-cook
  steak, e.g. rump, cut into
  32 x 2.5cm (1in) dice (all
  visible fat removed)

Combine the orange juice and half the orange zest, lime juice, garlic granules, Henderson's relish (or Worcestershire sauce), oregano, cumin (and chilli flakes and sweetener if using) in a bowl.

Add the diced steak to the marinade and mix until well coated. Cover and leave in the fridge for at least 1 hour (or overnight if you wish). Assemble the ingredients on eight skewers, alternating as follows: pepper, steak, onion, steak. Use four pieces of steak on each skewer.

Now, cook the rice. Place it in a pan and cover with 500ml cold water. Add a good pinch of salt and bring to the boil, then reduce the heat, cover, and simmer for 10 minutes until all the water has been absorbed. Remove from the heat, stir in the remaining orange zest and all the lime zest, cover and set aside while you cook the skewers.

Spray a griddle pan or heavy-based frying pan with low-calorie cooking spray and place over a high heat. When the pan is hot, place the

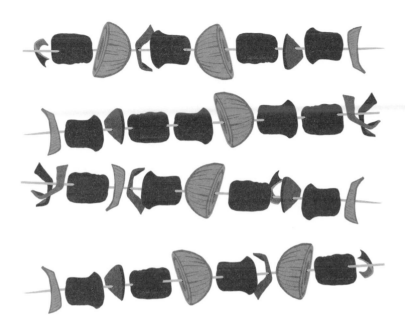

1 red pepper, halved, deseeded and cut into 8 x 2.5cm (1in) dice
1 small red onion, cut into 8 x 2.5cm (1in) dice
200g basmati rice
low-calorie cooking spray
4 spring onions, trimmed and sliced
10g fresh coriander leaves, chopped
rocket leaves, to serve

skewers in the pan and cook for 1 minute 30 seconds on each of the four sides. This should cook the steak to medium doneness. If you prefer it well done, cook the skewers for a little longer. You may need to do this in batches, depending on the size of your pan.

Stir the spring onions and coriander into the rice. Divide the rice among four plates, add two skewers to each plate, and serve with rocket leaves and lime wedges.

Tip

THESE ARE GREAT FOR A BARBECUE. IF USING BAMBOO SKEWERS, SOAK THEM IN WATER WHILE THE MEAT IS MARINATING, TO PREVENT THEM BURNING WHILE COOKING.

Day Five

BREAKFAST	VALUES
TOTAL	

LUNCH	VALUES
TOTAL	

DINNER	VALUES
TOTAL	

SNACKS AND TREATS	VALUES
TOTAL	

Notes

WATER

Day Six

BREAKFAST	VALUES
TOTAL	

LUNCH	VALUES
TOTAL	

DINNER	VALUES
TOTAL	

SNACKS AND TREATS	VALUES
TOTAL	

'I love recipes that are quick and simple to make, without needing to use lots of different ingredients; Mint Tea Lamb ticked all the boxes.' CAROLINE ISOBEL

WATER

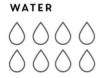

MINT TEA LAMB

🕐 **5 MINS*** | 🍲 **10 MINS** | ✕ **SERVES 2**

* PLUS MINIMUM 1 HOUR MARINATING AND 30 MINS RESTING

This might sound like a bizarre concept, but if you are a fan of lamb and mint sauce, then the dish might make more sense! Lamb and mint are the perfect combination, and by using mint tea bags to create a tasty marinade, you get that same great taste without the calories of a sweet sauce.

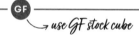

→ *use GF stock cube*

PER SERVING
320 KCAL
8.7G CARBS

2 mint tea bags, contents removed and bag discarded
1 lamb stock cube, crumbled
1 tbsp balsamic vinegar
300g lean lamb steaks or chops (240g once trimmed of visible fat)
80g frozen peas
120g broccoli, cut into small florets
low-calorie cooking spray
sea salt and freshly ground black pepper

In a small bowl or mug, mix the contents of the tea bags, the stock cube, balsamic vinegar and 3 tablespoons of boiling water until dissolved.

Put the lamb in a bowl and add the marinade. Coat the lamb in the marinade, cover, transfer to the fridge and leave to marinate for 1 hour, or even better overnight. (You can skip the marinating step if you are short of time, but it is worthwhile for the added flavour.)

Around 30 minutes before you wish to eat, remove the lamb from the fridge to bring the meat back to room temperature.

When you're ready to eat, put the peas and broccoli in a saucepan of boiling water and cook for 4–8 minutes, or until tender.

While the vegetables are cooking, spray a frying pan with low-calorie cooking spray and place over a medium heat. Add the lamb and pour over any remaining marinade. Cook the lamb for 4–5 minutes on each side (or longer

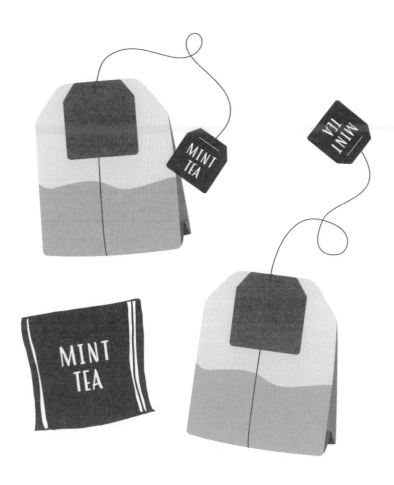

if you like your meat well done). Cut the meat near the centre to check it is cooked to your liking.

Tip
IF YOU DON'T HAVE ANY MINT TEA BAGS YOU CAN SUBSTITUTE WITH 2 TEASPOONS OF DRIED MINT.

When the vegetables are cooked, drain and season with salt and pepper. Serve the lamb with the vegetables, pouring any juices left in the pan over the meat.

WEEK 7

Day Seven

Tip
If you find breakfast difficult, prepare something the night before – such as overnight oats.

BREAKFAST	VALUES
TOTAL	

LUNCH	VALUES
TOTAL	

DINNER	VALUES
TOTAL	

SNACKS AND TREATS	VALUES
TOTAL	

Notes

WATER

○ ○ ○ ○
○ ○ ○ ○

Shopping List 1

....
....
....
....
....
....
....
....
....
....
....
....
....
....
....
....
....
....
....

Shopping List 2

....
....
....
....
....
....
....
....
....
....
....
....
....
....
....
....
....
....
....

Shopping List 2

....
....
....
....
....
....
....
....
....
....
....
....
....
....
....
....
....
....
....

Shopping List 1

....
....
....
....
....
....
....
....
....
....
....
....
....
....
....
....
....
....
....

YOU MAY NOT BE THERE YET BUT YOU'RE CLOSER than you WERE YESTERDAY

Eight

CHANGE +/-

CURRENT WEIGHT

THIS WEEK I WOULD LIKE TO ACHIEVE

LAST WEEK, THESE THINGS WENT WELL...

REMINDERS FOR THIS WEEK

◯ PLANNED MEALS

◯ SHOPPING DONE

◯ PLANNED EXERCISE

SPANISH EGGS

🕐 **15 MINS** | 🍲 **10–12 MINS** | ✕ **SERVES 2**

This tasty dish combines traditional Spanish flavours with rustic ingredients to make the perfect brunch. Using Quorn sausages means you can add a hint of classic chorizo flavouring, without the fat and calorie content. Serve it on its own, or to make a hearty lunch add a small bread roll or chunk of baguette for dunking!

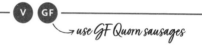

→ *use GF Quorn sausages*

PER SERVING
355 KCAL
27G CARBS

Equipment
2 x 16cm (6in) baking dishes

low-calorie cooking spray
3 Quorn sausages, sliced
  into 1cm (½in) pieces
75g Brussels sprouts,
  shredded
60g onion, finely diced
2 garlic cloves, crushed
1 tsp smoked paprika
1 x 400g tin cherry
  tomatoes
50g tinned borlotti beans
  (drained weight)
200g passata
2 medium eggs
chopped parsley leaves,
  to serve (optional)

Preheat the oven to 170°C (fan 150°C/gas mark 3).

Spray a frying pan with low-calorie cooking spray and place over a high heat. Fry the Quorn sausages, sprouts, onion and garlic for 3–4 minutes until lightly browned and the sprouts and onions have softened slightly.

Add all of the other ingredients to the frying pan, except the eggs, and mix well. Simmer over a medium heat for 2 minutes until bubbling gently.

Distribute the mixture between the two small baking dishes and make a small well in the top of each. Crack an egg into each well and bake in the oven for 8–10 minutes, until the egg white is cooked but the yolk is still runny.

Remove from the oven and serve straight away.

Tip
USE WHATEVER VEGETARIAN OR MEAT
SAUSAGES YOU LIKE – JUST REMEMBER
TO CHECK THE NUTRITIONAL VALUES OF
WHICHEVER YOU CHOOSE TO USE.

Weekly Meal Planner

	BREAKFAST	LUNCH
MONDAY		
TUESDAY		
WEDNESDAY		
THURSDAY		
FRIDAY		
SATURDAY		
SUNDAY		

Weekly Meal Planner

DINNER	SNACK	NOTES

Day One

BREAKFAST	VALUES
TOTAL	

LUNCH	VALUES
TOTAL	

DINNER	VALUES
TOTAL	

SNACKS AND TREATS	VALUES
TOTAL	

Notes

WATER

Day Two

BREAKFAST	VALUES
TOTAL	

LUNCH	VALUES
TOTAL	

DINNER	VALUES
TOTAL	

SNACKS AND TREATS	VALUES
TOTAL	

'Very tasty and easy to make, **Spanish Eggs** *make an excellent winter warmer*' **TARA**

WATER

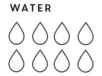

Day Three

BREAKFAST	VALUES
TOTAL	

LUNCH	VALUES
TOTAL	

DINNER	VALUES
TOTAL	

SNACKS AND TREATS	VALUES
TOTAL	

Notes

WATER

MUSHROOM STROGANOFF

🕐 **15 MINS** | 🍲 **15 MINS** | ✕ **SERVES 4**

A creamy, mustardy stroganoff sauce isn't only delicious with beef. Our vegetarian take on the Russian classic packs in the mushrooms, producing a rich dish that you would never believe is light on calories, or meat-free. The perfect vegetarian swap!

V **F** **GF**

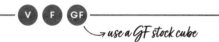 → use a GF stock cube

PER SERVING
338 KCAL
53G CARBS

200g basmati rice
sea salt
low-calorie cooking spray
1 onion, finely chopped
800g mushrooms, thickly
 sliced
4 garlic cloves, finely
 chopped or grated
1 tsp smoked paprika
½ tsp English mustard
 powder
100ml vegetable stock
 (1 vegetable stock cube
 dissolved in 100ml
 boiling water)
240g low-fat cream cheese
1 tbsp Henderson's relish
1 tsp white wine vinegar
10g fresh chives, finely
 chopped, to serve

Place the rice in a saucepan with 500ml cold water and a good pinch of salt. Bring to the boil, then reduce the heat, cover, and cook gently for 12–15 minutes, until all the water has been absorbed.

Meanwhile, make the stroganoff. Spray a large frying pan or wok with low-calorie cooking spray and place over a medium-high heat. Add the onion and mushrooms to the pan and sauté for 5 minutes. Add the garlic, paprika and mustard powder and cook for a further minute. Pour in the stock and stir in the cream cheese until it has softened and is well incorporated. Add the Henderson's relish and the vinegar. Bring to the boil and allow to bubble for 5–10 minutes until the sauce has thickened (how long it will take depends on the water content of the mushrooms). You could allow the sauce to cool at this point and freeze for another day.

Divide the rice among four plates, add the stroganoff and scatter with the chives.

Tip
SPICE UP YOUR STROGANOFF BY USING HOT SMOKED PAPRIKA, OR BY ADDING SOME CAYENNE PEPPER.

Day Four

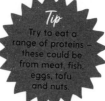

BREAKFAST	VALUES
TOTAL	

LUNCH	VALUES
TOTAL	

DINNER	VALUES
TOTAL	

SNACKS AND TREATS	VALUES
TOTAL	

Notes

WATER

○ ○ ○ ○
○ ○ ○ ○

Day Five

BREAKFAST	VALUES
TOTAL	

LUNCH	VALUES
TOTAL	

DINNER	VALUES
TOTAL	

SNACKS AND TREATS	VALUES
TOTAL	

Notes

_____

_____

_____

WATER

◇ ◇ ◇ ◇
◇ ◇ ◇ ◇

Day Six

BREAKFAST	VALUES
TOTAL	

LUNCH	VALUES
TOTAL	

DINNER	VALUES
TOTAL	

SNACKS AND TREATS	VALUES
TOTAL	

Notes

WATER

⬡ ⬡ ⬡ ⬡
⬡ ⬡ ⬡ ⬡

Day Seven

Week
EIGHT
done!

BREAKFAST	VALUES
TOTAL	

LUNCH	VALUES
TOTAL	

DINNER	VALUES
TOTAL	

SNACKS AND TREATS	VALUES
TOTAL	

'**Mushroom Stroganoff** *is hands
down one of my favourites.*'
MEGAN

WATER

○ ○ ○ ○
○ ○ ○ ○

WEEK
Nine

CHANGE +/-

CURRENT WEIGHT

THIS WEEK I WOULD LIKE TO ACHIEVE

LAST WEEK, THESE THINGS WENT WELL...

REMINDERS FOR THIS WEEK

○ PLANNED MEALS

○ SHOPPING DONE

○ PLANNED EXERCISE

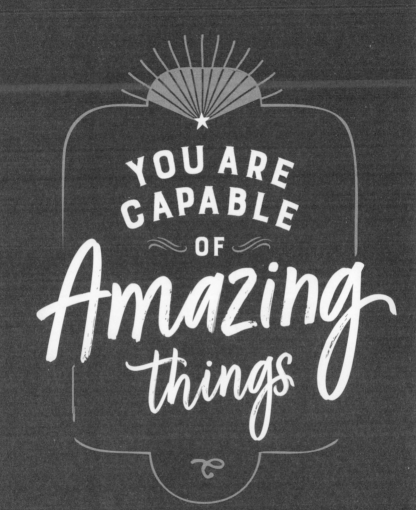

YOU ARE
CAPABLE
OF
Amazing
things

Weekly Meal Planner

	BREAKFAST	LUNCH
MONDAY		
TUESDAY		
WEDNESDAY		
THURSDAY		
FRIDAY		
SATURDAY		
SUNDAY		

Weekly Meal Planner

DINNER	SNACK	NOTES

Day One

BREAKFAST	VALUES
TOTAL	

LUNCH	VALUES
TOTAL	

DINNER	VALUES
TOTAL	

SNACKS AND TREATS	VALUES
TOTAL	

Notes

WATER

WEEK 9

Day Two

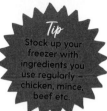

Tip
Stock up your freezer with ingredients you use regularly – chicken, mince, beef etc.

BREAKFAST	VALUES
TOTAL	

LUNCH	VALUES
TOTAL	

DINNER	VALUES
TOTAL	

SNACKS AND TREATS	VALUES
TOTAL	

Notes

WATER

○ ○ ○ ○
○ ○ ○ ○

133

Day Three

BREAKFAST	VALUES
TOTAL	

LUNCH	VALUES
TOTAL	

DINNER	VALUES
TOTAL	

SNACKS AND TREATS	VALUES
TOTAL	

> 'Wow! The **Veggie Shepherd's Pie** is a classic recipe that everyone can enjoy! Delicious, filling and really easy to make.'
> **CHARLENE**

WATER

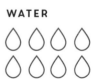

Day Four

BREAKFAST	VALUES
TOTAL	

LUNCH	VALUES
TOTAL	

DINNER	VALUES
TOTAL	

SNACKS AND TREATS	VALUES
TOTAL	

Notes

WATER

VEGGIE SHEPHERD'S PIE

🕐 **10 MINS** | 🍲 **55 MINS** | ✕ **SERVES 6**

It may be meat-free, but this veggie shepherd's pie – thanks to some clever seasoning – isn't short on flavour! Adding lentils and lots of lovely vegetables gives the dish filling power, making it a hearty dish for the whole family. It's also perfect for batch cooking, so you can plan ahead and feed the family easily if you're short on time.

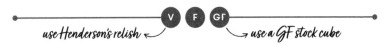

use Henderson's relish ← (V) (F) (GF) → *use a GF stock cube*

PER SERVING
375 KCAL
62G CARBS

low-calorie cooking spray
1 large celery stick, finely diced
1 large leek, trimmed and thinly sliced
2 carrots, finely diced
1 onion, finely diced
3 garlic cloves, minced
300g mushrooms, thinly sliced
2 x 400g tins green lentils, rinsed and drained
1 x 400g tin chopped tomatoes
1 tsp dried rosemary
1 tsp dried thyme
1 tsp Worcestershire sauce or Henderson's relish
1 tbsp balsamic vinegar
¼ tsp English mustard powder

Preheat the oven to 220°C (fan 200°C/gas mark 7).

Spray a large saucepan with low-calorie cooking spray and place over a medium heat. Add the celery, leek, carrot, onion and garlic and sauté for 10 minutes until the vegetables have softened and the onions are translucent.

Add the mushrooms, lentils, chopped tomatoes, rosemary, thyme, Worcestershire sauce, balsamic vinegar, mustard powder, red wine stock pot and vegetable stock to the pan. Bring to a simmer, then reduce the heat to low and simmer for 15 minutes while you prepare the mashed potatoes. Don't forget to stir it occasionally.

To make the mashed potato topping, bring a large saucepan of salted water to the boil. Add the potatoes and swede and cook for 10–15 minutes until tender – if you push a fork through the potatoes they should still hold their shape. Drain, then return to the pan.

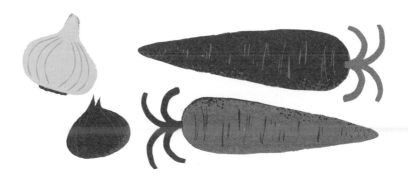

1 red wine stock pot
400ml vegetable stock
(1 vegetable stock cube
dissolved in 400ml boiling
water)
2 tbsp tomato puree
150g frozen peas

FOR THE MASHED
POTATO TOPPING

1kg potatoes, peeled and
cut into 3cm (1¼ in) cubes
1 large swede, peeled and
cut into 1cm (½ in) cubes
¼ tsp English mustard
powder
1 medium egg, whisked
sea salt and freshly ground
black pepper

Mash the potatoes and swede until smooth and fluffy. Add the mustard powder and egg and season with salt and pepper. Mash until combined and set aside.

Stir the tomato puree and frozen peas into the lentil mixture and season with salt and pepper, then pour the mix into the bottom of a large roasting dish or pie dish.

Spread the mashed potato and swede evenly over the top of the lentil mixture, drag a fork over the surface of the mash (this will help the topping crisp up). (The unbaked pie can be frozen once cooled and cooked from frozen.)

Place the pie into the centre of the oven. Bake for 30 minutes, until the mash is golden at the edges.

Remove from the oven and serve. The pie can also be frozen once cooled.

Tips

• MAKE IT VEGAN BY USING HENDERSON'S RELISH AND LEAVING THE EGG OUT OF THE MASH.

• FOR SUPER-CREAMY POTATOES ADD A LITTLE SPLASH OF WATER AND USE AN ELECTRIC WHISK AFTER MASHING.

Day Five

BREAKFAST	VALUES
TOTAL	

LUNCH	VALUES
TOTAL	

DINNER	VALUES
TOTAL	

SNACKS AND TREATS	VALUES
TOTAL	

Notes

WATER

Day Six

BREAKFAST

	VALUES
TOTAL	

LUNCH

	VALUES
TOTAL	

DINNER

	VALUES
TOTAL	

SNACKS AND TREATS

	VALUES
TOTAL	

*The **Veggie Shepherd's Pie** is a very tasty alternative to a meat one. Lovely flavours. Would definitely make it again.'*
SHIRLEY

WATER

HUNTERS' CHICKEN LASAGNE

🕐 **15 MINS** | 🍲 **60 MINS** | ✕ **SERVES 4**

A combination of two favourite comfort dishes, this Hunters'
Chicken Lasagne feels like an indulgence but the move away from
full-fat butter and cheese-laden white sauce keeps this recipe
everyday light. Watch as the cheese bubbles and turns golden in
the oven; this meal is so tasty and a winner for everyone!

PER SERVING
383 KCAL
38.7G CARBS

low-calorie cooking spray
400g chicken breast, cut
 into small 1cm (½in)
 chunks
1 medium onion, peeled
 and diced
2 green peppers, deseeded
 and diced
1 tbsp smoked paprika
1½ tsp garlic granules
¼ tsp chilli powder
2 tbsp tomato puree
1 x 400g tin chopped
 tomatoes
200ml chicken stock
 (1 chicken stock
 cube dissolved in
 200ml boiling water)
2 tbsp balsamic vinegar
1 tbsp Worcestershire
 sauce or Henderson's relish
6 lasagne sheets

Preheat the oven to 180°C (fan 160°C/gas mark 4).

Spray a large saucepan or wok with low-calorie
cooking spray. Sauté the chicken over a medium
heat for 3–4 minutes, until sealed. Add the onion
and peppers and stir well. Add the paprika,
garlic granules and chilli powder, then stir in the
tomato puree and cook for a minute. Pour in the
chopped tomatoes and chicken stock. Add the
balsamic vinegar and Worcestershire sauce. Stir
well and bring to a simmer. Cook for 10 minutes.

Next, prepare the topping. Cut the bacon
medallions into small 5mm (¼in) pieces.
Beat together the yoghurt and egg. Add
2 tablespoons of cold water. Stir in the bacon
and season with salt and pepper, remembering
that the bacon will be a little salty.

Now, assemble the lasagne. Pour half of the
chicken mix into a deep lasagne dish. Top with
three sheets of lasagne. Pour over the rest of
the chicken mixture, then place the rest of the
lasagne sheets on top.

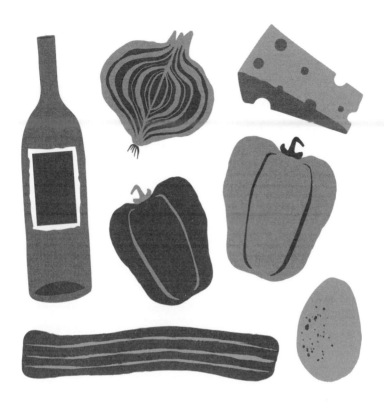

FOR THE TOPPING

2 bacon medallions
250g fat-free Greek-style
   yoghurt
1 medium egg
sea salt and freshly ground
   black pepper
30g reduced-fat cheese,
   finely grated

TO ACCOMPANY
(*optional*)

75g mixed side salad
   (+ 15 kcal per serving)

Pour over the topping and sprinkle over the cheese. Place in the oven and cook for 40 minutes, until a knife slides easily into the middle. Serve with a crispy side salad, if you like. (Lasagne freezes well, so you can also cool it and keep it to have another day – defrost thoroughly before reheating.)

Day Seven

BREAKFAST	VALUES
TOTAL	

LUNCH	VALUES
TOTAL	

DINNER	VALUES
TOTAL	

SNACKS AND TREATS	VALUES
TOTAL	

Notes

WATER

Shopping List 1

....
....
....
....
....
....
....
....
....
....
....
....
....
....
....
....
....
....

Shopping List 2

....
....
....
....
....
....
....
....
....
....
....
....
....
....
....
....
....

Shopping List ❷

....
....
....
....
....
....
....
....
....
....
....
....
....
....
....
....
....
....

Shopping List ❶

....
....
....
....
....
....
....
....
....
....
....
....
....
....
....
....
....
....

EVERY NEW DAY *is* a chance to CHANGE *your* LIFE

Ten

CHANGE +/-

CURRENT WEIGHT

THIS WEEK I WOULD LIKE TO ACHIEVE

LAST WEEK, THESE THINGS WENT WELL...

REMINDERS FOR THIS WEEK

○ PLANNED MEALS

○ SHOPPING DONE

○ PLANNED EXERCISE

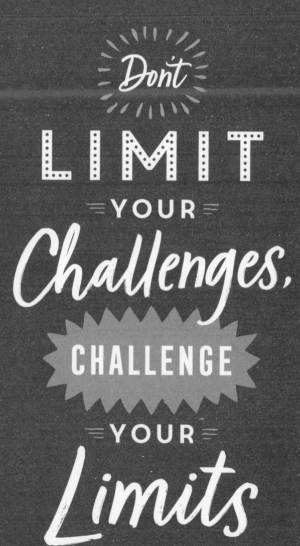

Don't
LIMIT
YOUR
Challenges,
CHALLENGE
YOUR
Limits

Weekly Meal Planner

	BREAKFAST	LUNCH
MONDAY		
TUESDAY		
WEDNESDAY		
THURSDAY		
FRIDAY		
SATURDAY		
SUNDAY		

Weekly Meal Planner

DINNER	SNACK	NOTES

WEEK 10
Day One

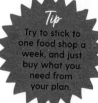

Tip
Try to stick to one food shop a week, and just buy what you need from your plan.

BREAKFAST	VALUES
TOTAL	

LUNCH	VALUES
TOTAL	

DINNER	VALUES
TOTAL	

SNACKS AND TREATS	VALUES
TOTAL	

Notes

WATER

◇ ◇ ◇ ◇
◇ ◇ ◇ ◇

Day Two

BREAKFAST	VALUES
TOTAL	

LUNCH	VALUES
TOTAL	

DINNER	VALUES
TOTAL	

SNACKS AND TREATS	VALUES
TOTAL	

Notes

WATER

◇ ◇ ◇ ◇
◇ ◇ ◇ ◇

MANGO *and* CHILLI CHICKEN FLATTIES

🕐 **10 MINS*** | 🍲 **15 MINS** | ✕ **SERVES 4**

* PLUS MINIMUM 1 HOUR MARINATING

This simple chicken recipe brings the flavours and colours of summer to a meal that can be enjoyed on any day of the year. The mango ketchup is a great way of using up the excess marinade: making it into a dipping sauce gives the chicken extra fruitiness! Serve with rice or a side salad.

SERVES 4
161 KCAL
8.9G CARBS

150g fresh mango
juice of 1 lime
1 garlic clove, crushed
1 fresh red chilli, deseeded
sea salt and freshly ground
   black pepper
2 x 200g skinless chicken
   breasts
low-calorie cooking spray
200ml water
1 tsp cider vinegar
2 tbsp tomato puree
1 tsp granulated sweetener

TO ACCOMPANY
(optional)
125g cooked rice per
   portion (+ 173 kcal
   per serving)

Place the mango, lime juice, crushed garlic and red chilli in a food processor. Season with a little salt and pepper and blitz for a few seconds until the chilli is finely chopped and the mango is almost smooth. Transfer to a wide, shallow dish and set aside.

Slice the chicken breasts horizontally into 'steaks' about 1.5cm (¾ in) thick. Place the chicken pieces in the blitzed mango mixture, cover, and leave in the fridge to marinate for at least 1 hour, or overnight.

Spray a large frying pan with some low-calorie cooking spray and place over a medium heat. Add the marinated chicken 'flatties' to the frying pan, setting aside the leftover marinade. Fry for 4–5 minutes, until golden, then turn over the chicken pieces and cook for another 3–4 minutes until golden on both sides and cooked through. Remove from the frying pan and keep warm.

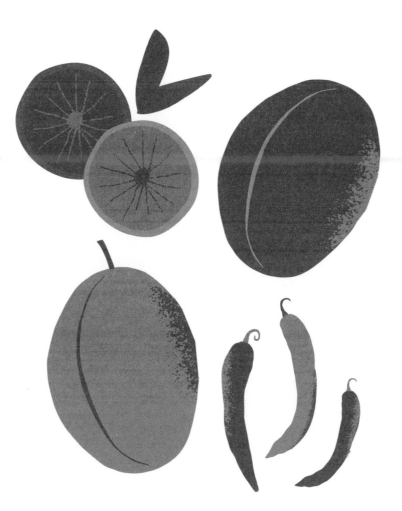

Tips

• **IF YOU PREFER YOUR FOOD WITH A STRONGER KICK, ADD A DASH OF HOT CHILLI SAUCE TO THE MARINADE.**

• **THESE FLATTIES COULD BE COOKED ON THE BARBECUE.**

To make the mango ketchup, return the frying pan to the heat and add the leftover marinade, plus the remaining ingredients. Stir and reduce over a high heat for 5–6 minutes until piping hot and thickened.

Serve the chicken flatties with the mango ketchup for dipping! They can be frozen once cooled.

Day Three

BREAKFAST	VALUES
TOTAL	

LUNCH	VALUES
TOTAL	

DINNER	VALUES
TOTAL	

SNACKS AND TREATS	VALUES
TOTAL	

Notes

WATER

○ ○ ○ ○
○ ○ ○ ○

Day Four

BREAKFAST	VALUES
TOTAL	

LUNCH	VALUES
TOTAL	

DINNER	VALUES
TOTAL	

SNACKS AND TREATS	VALUES
TOTAL	

'The **Mango and Chilli Chicken Flatties** are AMAZING! What a stunner of a recipe.' **HARRIET**

WATER

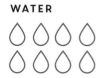

BURRITOS

🕐 **10 MINS** | 🍲 **40 MINS** | ✕ **SERVES 6**

Nothing beats a burrito. We've lightened up this classic wrap by leaving out the rice and instead packing it full of extra-tasty beans and veggies. Leaving out the rice means there's even more room for the gooey cheese, garlic sauce and tender pulled chicken. That's our kind of burrito!

PER SERVING
339 KCAL
34G CARBS

2 large skinless chicken breasts
300ml chicken stock (1 chicken stock cube dissolved in 300ml boiling water)
1 tsp garlic granules
½ tsp chilli powder
juice of 1 lime
3 tomatoes, finely diced
1 red pepper, halved, deseeded and diced
1 red onion, finely diced
1 x 400g tin black beans, drained and rinsed
1 x 200g tin sweetcorn, drained
handful of fresh coriander, roughly chopped
¼ tsp sweet smoked paprika
sea salt and freshly ground black pepper

Preheat the oven to 220°C (fan 200°C/gas mark 7).

Put the chicken breasts in a roasting dish, pour over the stock, add half the garlic granules, the chilli powder and half the lime juice, stir and place in the oven. Bake for 40 minutes.

While the chicken is cooking, mix the diced tomatoes in a bowl with the red pepper, onion, black beans, sweetcorn, coriander, paprika and the remaining lime juice. Season to taste with salt and pepper and place in the fridge.

Mix the yoghurt in a bowl with the remaining garlic granules. Place in the fridge.

When the chicken is cooked through, remove it from the roasting dish and shred the meat with two forks (keep the oven on). Pour over 3 tablespoons of the remaining stock to keep the meat moist.

Take a tortilla and spoon some of the vegetable and bean mix, pulled chicken, garlic-yoghurt

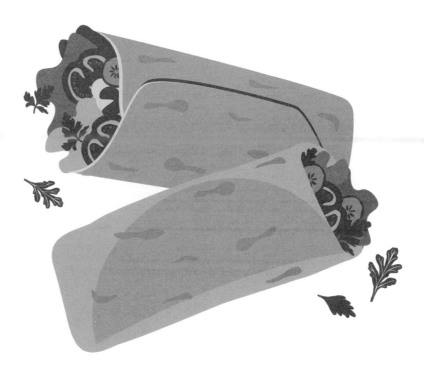

100g fat-free Greek-style yoghurt
6 low-calorie tortilla wraps
120g reduced-fat Cheddar, finely grated

Tips

• **YOU CAN MAKE ALL THE ELEMENTS OF THE BURRITOS IN ADVANCE, READY TO ASSEMBLE AT DINNER TIME.**

• **IF YOU LIKE HOT SPICE, ADD SOME CHILLI POWDER TO THE VEGETABLE AND BEAN MIX.**

sauce and grated cheese into the middle. Fold in both ends and tightly roll the tortilla to form a burrito.

Place the burrito onto a piece of foil larger than the tortilla. Tightly roll the burrito up in the foil and twist the ends like a cracker. Repeat with the rest of the tortillas.

Place the foil-wrapped burritos on a baking tray and place in the oven for 5 minutes, until piping hot throughout.

Remove from the oven and serve.

Day Five

BREAKFAST	VALUES
TOTAL	

LUNCH	VALUES
TOTAL	

DINNER	VALUES
TOTAL	

SNACKS AND TREATS	VALUES
TOTAL	

Notes

WATER

○ ○ ○ ○
○ ○ ○ ○

WEEK 10

Day Six

BREAKFAST		VALUES
	TOTAL	

LUNCH		VALUES
	TOTAL	

DINNER		VALUES
	TOTAL	

SNACKS AND TREATS		VALUES
	TOTAL	

"The Burritos went down so well! The freshness of having it with extra beans and other veg instead of rice is just lush! I can see it being a firm favourite on our menu.'

CHARLI MARIE

WATER

Day Seven

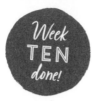

Week
TEN
done!

BREAKFAST	VALUES
TOTAL	

LUNCH	VALUES
TOTAL	

DINNER	VALUES
TOTAL	

SNACKS AND TREATS	VALUES
TOTAL	

Notes

WATER

○ ○ ○ ○
○ ○ ○ ○

WAKE
· UP ·
Kick Ass
Repeat

Eleven

CHANGE +/-

CURRENT WEIGHT

THIS WEEK I WOULD LIKE TO ACHIEVE

LAST WEEK, THESE THINGS WENT WELL...

REMINDERS FOR THIS WEEK

◯ **PLANNED MEALS**

◯ **SHOPPING DONE**

◯ **PLANNED EXERCISE**

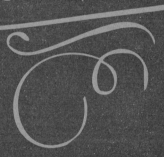

· BE YOUR OWN ·

cheerleader

BARBECUE KIEVS

🕐 **15 MINS** | 🍲 **30 MINS** | ✕ **SERVES 4**

Our twist on the classic chicken Kiev throws the usual garlic butter combo out of the window and instead combines barbecue flavours with gooey cheese and crispy breadcrumbs ... what's not to like?! The liquid smoke can be found in most supermarkets among the condiments and sauces. It makes the sauce taste like a proper barbecue sauce, but it can totally be made without it, too.

F GF

→ use GF breadcrumbs

PER SERVING
307 KCAL
12G CARBS

4 x 200g skinless chicken breasts
2 mini 'light' Babybel cheeses
60g wholemeal bread, blitzed into fine crumbs
low-calorie cooking spray

FOR THE BARBECUE SAUCE
200g passata
1 tbsp granulated sweetener
1 tbsp Worcestershire sauce
2 tbsp cider vinegar
2 tsp liquid smoke (optional)
1 tsp garlic granules
½ tsp smoked paprika
¼ tsp English mustard powder

TO ACCOMPANY *(optional)*
75g mixed side salad
(+ 15 kcal per serving)

Preheat the oven to 180°C (fan 160°C/gas mark 4) and line a baking tray with baking parchment.

Place all of the barbecue sauce ingredients in a saucepan and bring to a simmer over a medium heat. Cook for 10 minutes until the sauce has reduced by half, then set aside.

Prepare the chicken by cutting a large pocket in one end of the chicken breast (along the 'short' edge), being careful not to pierce the outside of the chicken. Cut the Babybels in half crossways through the middle.

Place a piece of cheese into each pocket in the chicken breasts and feed in as much of the barbecue sauce as possible.

Place the breadcrumbs in a shallow dish and spread a little of the remaining barbecue sauce all over each chicken breast. Dip each piece of chicken into the breadcrumbs to coat lightly and place them on the lined baking tray. (You

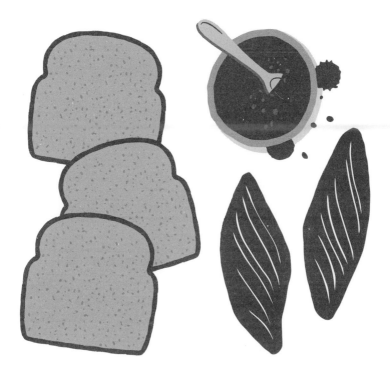

could freeze the chicken Kievs at this point to thoroughly defrost and cook on another day.)

Spray the breasts with low-calorie cooking spray and transfer to the oven.

Bake the chicken for 15 minutes, then turn over each chicken breast, spray with more low-calorie cooking spray and sprinkle any leftover breadcrumbs from the shallow dish on top. Cook for a further 15 minutes until the chicken is cooked through and the cheese has melted.

Remove from the oven and serve with a mixed salad (if you like). The baked Kievs can be frozen once cooled – defrost thoroughly before reheating.

Tips

• USE A COCKTAIL STICK TO HOLD THE CHICKEN BREASTS TOGETHER ONCE FILLED, IF REQUIRED.

• KEEP BACK SOME BARBECUE SAUCE (BEING CAREFUL NOT TO CONTAMINATE IT WITH RAW CHICKEN) TO USE AS A DIP FOR YOUR KIEVS.

Weekly Meal Planner

	BREAKFAST	LUNCH
MONDAY		
TUESDAY		
WEDNESDAY		
THURSDAY		
FRIDAY		
SATURDAY		
SUNDAY		

Weekly Meal Planner

DINNER	SNACK	NOTES

Day One

BREAKFAST	VALUES
TOTAL	

LUNCH	VALUES
TOTAL	

DINNER	VALUES
TOTAL	

SNACKS AND TREATS	VALUES
TOTAL	

Notes

WATER

○ ○ ○ ○
○ ○ ○ ○

Day Two

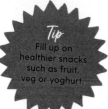

BREAKFAST	VALUES
TOTAL	

LUNCH	VALUES
TOTAL	

DINNER	VALUES
TOTAL	

SNACKS AND TREATS	VALUES
TOTAL	

Notes

WATER

○ ○ ○ ○
○ ○ ○ ○

Day Three

BREAKFAST	VALUES
TOTAL	

LUNCH	VALUES
TOTAL	

DINNER	VALUES
TOTAL	

SNACKS AND TREATS	VALUES
TOTAL	

> 'The **Barbecue Kievs**
> are blooming amazing!
> *FAB-U-LOUS.*' **HELEN**

WATER

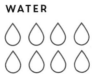

Day Four

BREAKFAST	VALUES
TOTAL	

LUNCH	VALUES
TOTAL	

DINNER	VALUES
TOTAL	

SNACKS AND TREATS	VALUES
TOTAL	

Notes

WATER

FULLY-LOADED BACON FRIES

🕐 **5 MINS** | 🍲 **45 MINS** | ✗ **SERVES 4**

This pile of tasty fries covered in gooey cheese, crispy bacon and a sweet and smoky sauce is inspired by those delicious but oh-so-naughty sides in gourmet burger restaurants. We can't think of anything better than fries, bacon, garlic and cheese, and you won't believe it but this dish is slimming friendly!

 GF

PER SERVING
342 KCAL
47G CARBS

low-calorie cooking spray
1kg potatoes, scrubbed clean (skin left on) and cut into 5mm (¼ in)-thick fries
½ tsp garlic granules
120g smoked bacon medallions, cut into small pieces (or use unsmoked if you prefer)
80g reduced-fat Cheddar, finely grated
2 spring onions, trimmed and thinly sliced

Tip
THE STRONGER THE CHEDDAR THE BETTER WITH THIS DISH.

Preheat the oven to 220°C (fan 200°/gas mark 7). Line a large baking tray with foil and spray with low-calorie cooking spray.

Place the fries on the lined tray, spray with low-calorie cooking spray and sprinkle over the garlic granules. Toss until evenly coated. Spread the fries out on the tray (use a second baking tray lined with foil and sprayed with cooking spray if the fries are too crowded on a single tray).

Place the fries in the middle of the oven and bake for 30 minutes, then carefully turn them over and re-spray with low-calorie cooking spray before placing back in the oven for a further 10 minutes, or until cooked through and crispy on the outside.

While the fries are cooking, place a frying pan over a medium heat, spray with low-calorie cooking spray, add the bacon pieces and fry until crispy. Remove from the heat and set to one side.

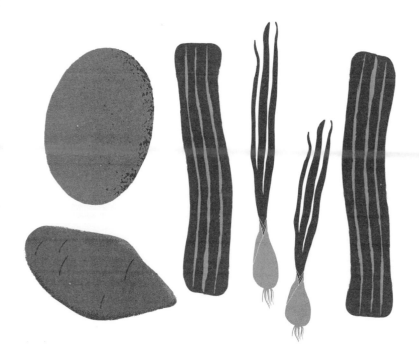

FOR THE SAUCE

¼ tsp garlic granules
150g fat-free Greek-style yoghurt
1 tsp sweet smoked paprika
¼ tsp onion granules
1 tbsp balsamic vinegar

TO ACCOMPANY
(optional)

75g mixed side salad
(+ 15 kcal per serving)

To make the sauce, mix together the garlic granules, yoghurt, paprika, onion granules and balsamic vinegar in a bowl until smooth. It should be a similar thickness to ketchup (you may need to add a little cold water to loosen it if the Greek yoghurt is very thick). Place in the fridge until the fries are done.

Once the fries are cooked, transfer them to an ovenproof dish (choose one you're happy to serve the loaded fries in). Sprinkle over the grated cheese and the cooked bacon bits. Place the dish in the oven for a few minutes until the cheese has melted.

Once the cheese has melted, remove the dish from the oven and drizzle over the sauce, then serve with the sliced spring onions sprinkled on top.

Day Five

BREAKFAST	VALUES
TOTAL	

LUNCH	VALUES
TOTAL	

DINNER	VALUES
TOTAL	

SNACKS AND TREATS	VALUES
TOTAL	

Notes

WATER

○ ○ ○ ○
○ ○ ○ ○

Day Six

BREAKFAST	VALUES
TOTAL	

LUNCH	VALUES
TOTAL	

DINNER	VALUES
TOTAL	

SNACKS AND TREATS	VALUES
TOTAL	

'Amazing! The **Fully-Loaded Bacon Fries** are a tasty treat for all the family.' **SARAH**

WATER

WEEK 11

Day Seven

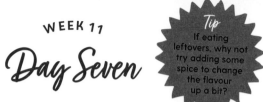

Tip
If eating leftovers, why not try adding some spice to change the flavour up a bit?

BREAKFAST	VALUES
TOTAL	

LUNCH	VALUES
TOTAL	

DINNER	VALUES
TOTAL	

SNACKS AND TREATS	VALUES
TOTAL	

Notes

WATER

◇ ◇ ◇ ◇
◇ ◇ ◇ ◇

176

Shopping List 1

....
....
....
....
....
....
....
....
....
....
....
....
....
....
....
....
....
....
....

Shopping List 2

....
....
....
....
....
....
....
....
....
....
....
....
....
....
....
....
....
....

Shopping List ②

....
....
....
....
....
....
....
....
....
....
....
....
....
....
....
....
....
....
....

Shopping List ①

....
....
....
....
....
....
....
....
....
....
....
....
....
....
....
....
....
....

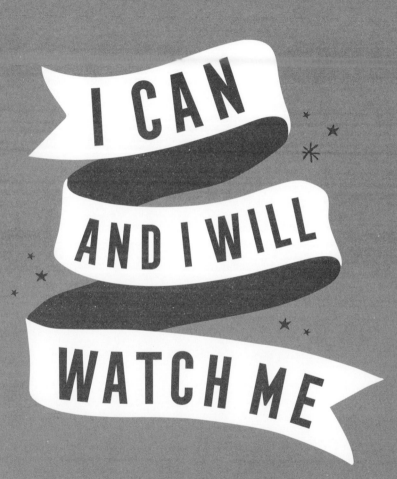

Twelve

CHANGE +/-

CURRENT WEIGHT

THIS WEEK I WOULD LIKE TO ACHIEVE

LAST WEEK, THESE THINGS WENT WELL...

REMINDERS FOR THIS WEEK

○ PLANNED MEALS

○ SHOPPING DONE

○ PLANNED EXERCISE

MEXICAN-STYLE BABY CORN

🕐 **5 MINS** | 🍲 **20 MINS** | ✕ **SERVES 2**

This tasty little side dish is inspired by grilled Mexican street corn (also known as elote). We've replaced corn on the cob with roasted baby corn, but kept the creamy cheese topping, which has a hint of spice and citrus to balance the sweet, delicious corn.

PER SERVING
94 KCAL
9.7G CARBS

260g baby corn
low-calorie cooking spray
¼ tsp chilli powder, plus extra to serve
¼ tsp garlic granules
small handful of fresh coriander, chopped
2 lime wedges, to serve

FOR THE SAUCE
40g fat-free Greek-style yoghurt
¼ tsp smoked paprika
20g reduced-fat feta cheese, crumbled
sea salt and freshly ground black pepper

Preheat the oven to 220°C (fan 200°C/gas mark 7).

Place the baby corn in a roasting dish, spray with low-calorie cooking spray and toss until coated.

Season the corn with the chilli powder and garlic granules and place in the oven. Bake for 20 minutes, until the corn has softened and browned at the edges but still has some bite.

While the corn is cooking, mix the yoghurt in a bowl with the paprika and crumbled feta. Season with salt and pepper to taste, then set aside until the corn is ready.

Remove the corn from the oven. Spread the yoghurt mix on top of the corn and sprinkle over the chopped coriander and a pinch of chilli powder. Serve with a wedge of lime to squeeze over.

IF YOU PREFER, YOU CAN MAKE THIS DISH USING TWO FULL-SIZE CORN ON THE COB INSTEAD (124 KCAL PER SERVING).

Weekly Meal Planner

	BREAKFAST	LUNCH
MONDAY		
TUESDAY		
WEDNESDAY		
THURSDAY		
FRIDAY		
SATURDAY		
SUNDAY		

Weekly Meal Planner

DINNER	SNACK	NOTES

YOU CAN'T GO
BACK AND CHANGE
THE BEGINNING
BUT YOU CAN
START WHERE YOU
ARE AND CHANGE
THE ENDING

Day One

BREAKFAST	VALUES
TOTAL	

LUNCH	VALUES
TOTAL	

DINNER	VALUES
TOTAL	

SNACKS AND TREATS	VALUES
TOTAL	

Notes

WATER

Day Two

BREAKFAST	VALUES
TOTAL	

LUNCH	VALUES
TOTAL	

DINNER	VALUES
TOTAL	

SNACKS AND TREATS	VALUES
TOTAL	

Notes

WATER

◊ ◊ ◊ ◊
◊ ◊ ◊ ◊

Day Three

BREAKFAST	VALUES
TOTAL	

LUNCH	VALUES
TOTAL	

DINNER	VALUES
TOTAL	

SNACKS AND TREATS	VALUES
TOTAL	

'Mexican-style Baby Corn *is a game changer. The sauce is just the right amount of spice and sour to go with the sweetcorn. Will definitely be making it again.'* JOZI

WATER

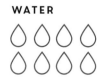

CARIBBEAN-STYLE CHICKEN *and* RICE SALAD

🕐 **15 MINS** | 🍲 **20 MINS** | ✖ **SERVES 4**

This salad is so tasty: it will feel like you're having a holiday meal in the middle of the week! The protein-rich chicken keeps you feeling full and satisfied, while the Caribbean seasoning adds a huge hit of flavour – it's a perfect combo. And mild spicing and sweet pineapple are just so good together. Get out that beach chair and enjoy!

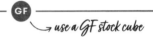

GF → *use a GF stock cube*

PER SERVING
392 KCAL
50G CARBS

low-calorie cooking spray
4 small, skinless chicken breasts
1 tbsp Jerk seasoning
1 lime, halved, plus extra wedges to serve
200g basmati rice
500ml chicken stock (1 chicken stock cube dissolved in 500ml boiling water)
3–4 sprigs of thyme
¼ tsp ground turmeric
1 medium red pepper, halved, deseeded and chopped
4 spring onions, trimmed and chopped

Preheat the oven to 180°C (fan 160°C/gas mark 4) and spray a baking tray with low-calorie cooking spray.

Coat the chicken breasts with the Jerk seasoning and place on the baking tray. Squeeze the juice of half the lime over the chicken, then place in the oven and cook for 15–20 minutes, until the juices run clear when the breasts are pierced with a knife, and there is no pink left in the middle.

While the chicken is cooking, place the rice in a saucepan, pour over the stock, and add the sprigs of thyme and the turmeric. Bring to the boil, then reduce the heat, cover, and simmer for 15 minutes, or until all the stock has been absorbed and the rice is cooked. Remove the thyme sprigs and transfer the rice to a large mixing bowl to cool.

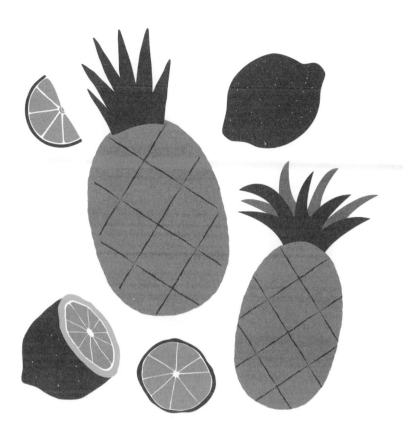

1 x 200g tin sweetcorn,
  drained (160g drained
  weight)
150g fresh pineapple,
  chopped
25g rocket leaves, roughly
  chopped

When the rice is cool, stir through the pepper,
spring onions, sweetcorn, pineapple and rocket,
and squeeze over the remaining lime.

Slice the chicken. Divide the rice salad among
four plates or bowls, and top with the sliced
chicken. Serve with lime wedges.

Tip
**THIS IS A GREAT
DISH FOR PACKED
LUNCHES.**

Day Four

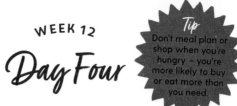

BREAKFAST	VALUES
TOTAL	

LUNCH	VALUES
TOTAL	

DINNER	VALUES
TOTAL	

SNACKS AND TREATS	VALUES
TOTAL	

Notes

WATER

◇ ◇ ◇ ◇
◇ ◇ ◇ ◇

Day Five

BREAKFAST	VALUES
TOTAL	

LUNCH	VALUES
TOTAL	

DINNER	VALUES
TOTAL	

SNACKS AND TREATS	VALUES
TOTAL	

Notes

WATER

Day Six

BREAKFAST	VALUES
TOTAL	

LUNCH	VALUES
TOTAL	

DINNER	VALUES
TOTAL	

SNACKS AND TREATS	VALUES
TOTAL	

Notes

WATER

Day Seven

BREAKFAST	VALUES
TOTAL	

LUNCH	VALUES
TOTAL	

DINNER	VALUES
TOTAL	

SNACKS AND TREATS	VALUES
TOTAL	

'I love the flavours in the **Caribbean-style Chicken and Rice Salad** – *so fresh and zingy.*'
VIENNA

WATER

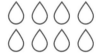

Thirteen

CHANGE +/-

CURRENT WEIGHT

THIS WEEK I WOULD LIKE TO ACHIEVE

LAST WEEK, THESE THINGS WENT WELL...

REMINDERS FOR THIS WEEK

○ PLANNED
MEALS

○ SHOPPING
DONE

○ PLANNED
EXERCISE

CHEESY CHILLI BEAN POT

🕐 **15 MINS** | 🍲 **30 MINS** | ✕ **SERVES 4**

This vegetarian chilli is rich with pasta and cheese and flavourful veg and beans. All your favourite warming foods, in a quick, easy and comforting one-pot dish. Don't worry if you're not a fan of hot spices; you can adjust the amount of chilli powder to keep it mild or spice it up – the choice is yours!

PER SERVING
395 KCAL
55G CARBS

low-calorie cooking spray
1 medium onion, diced
1 medium red pepper, halved, deseeded and diced
1 medium courgette, diced
4 garlic cloves, minced
1 tsp chilli powder (use more if you like it spicy)
1 tsp ground cumin
1 tsp dried oregano
1 x 400g tin chopped tomatoes
1 tbsp Henderson's relish
450ml vegetable stock (2 vegetable stock cubes dissolved in 450ml boiling water)
2 x 400g tins mixed beans, drained and rinsed
150g small pasta shapes (e.g. macaroni, fusilli, penne)
60g reduced-fat mature Cheddar, grated
10g fresh coriander leaves, chopped

Spray a large, heavy-based saucepan with low-calorie cooking spray and place over a medium heat. Add the onion, pepper and courgette and sauté for 3–4 minutes until the vegetables are beginning to soften, then add the garlic, spices and dried oregano to the pan and stir for a further minute, to allow the spices to release their flavours.

Add the chopped tomatoes and Henderson's relish and stir in the stock. When it starts to bubble, reduce the heat, cover and simmer for 10 minutes.

Stir in the drained beans and the pasta. (You can add a little water at this stage if you would like a looser sauce.) Replace the lid and continue cooking for a further 15 minutes.

When the pasta is cooked, stir in the cheese and the chopped coriander, and serve.

Tip
THIS DISH CAN BE FROZEN ONCE COOKED, BEFORE ADDING THE CHEESE AND CORIANDER.

Weekly Meal Planner

	BREAKFAST	LUNCH
MONDAY		
TUESDAY		
WEDNESDAY		
THURSDAY		
FRIDAY		
SATURDAY		
SUNDAY		

Weekly Meal Planner

DINNER	SNACK	NOTES

Day One

BREAKFAST	VALUES
TOTAL	

LUNCH	VALUES
TOTAL	

DINNER	VALUES
TOTAL	

SNACKS AND TREATS	VALUES
TOTAL	

Notes

WATER

◊ ◊ ◊ ◊
◊ ◊ ◊ ◊

Day Two

BREAKFAST	VALUES
TOTAL	

LUNCH	VALUES
TOTAL	

DINNER	VALUES
TOTAL	

SNACKS AND TREATS	VALUES
TOTAL	

'The **Cheesy Chilli Bean Pot** is very tasty! Extremely quick and easy to make. Perfect for lunches.'

NIAMH

WATER

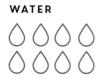

Day Three

BREAKFAST	VALUES
TOTAL	

LUNCH	VALUES
TOTAL	

DINNER	VALUES
TOTAL	

SNACKS AND TREATS	VALUES
TOTAL	

Notes

WATER

WEEK 13

Day Four

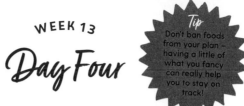

Tip
Don't ban foods from your plan – having a little of what you fancy can really help you to stay on track!

BREAKFAST	VALUES
TOTAL	

LUNCH	VALUES
TOTAL	

DINNER	VALUES
TOTAL	

SNACKS AND TREATS	VALUES
TOTAL	

Notes

_____

_____

_____

_____

WATER

○ ○ ○ ○
○ ○ ○ ○

Day Five

BREAKFAST	VALUES
TOTAL	

LUNCH	VALUES
TOTAL	

DINNER	VALUES
TOTAL	

SNACKS AND TREATS	VALUES
TOTAL	

'Wow – the **Chicken Forestiere** was lovely and so easy to make.' **DEBBIE**

WATER

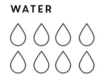

CHICKEN FORESTIERE

🕐 **10 MINS** | 🍲 **20 MINS** | ✗ **SERVES 4**

This succulent chicken breast dish, with its woodland flavours of mushrooms, garlic and thyme, will transport you to a small French town square, sharing a large, hearty family meal. But this is, of course, a more slimming-friendly twist on the French classic.

F **GF** 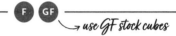 → *use GF stock cubes*

PER SERVING
212 KCAL
5.5G CARBS

low-calorie cooking spray
4 skinless chicken breasts
2 bacon medallions, cut
   into small pieces
150g shallots, finely chopped
300g mushrooms, sliced
2 garlic cloves, finely
   chopped or grated
10g fresh thyme leaves,
   chopped
300ml chicken stock
   (2 chicken stock cubes
   dissolved in 300ml
   boiling water)
1 tsp white wine vinegar
60g reduced-fat,
   spreadable cheese
freshly ground black
   pepper

TO ACCOMPANY
(optional)
Baby Roasties, page 71
   (+ 178 kcal per serving)

Spray a large, heavy-based shallow non-stick pan with low-calorie cooking spray and place over a high heat. Place the chicken breasts in the pan and brown for 2 minutes on each side, then remove from the pan and set to one side.

Reduce the heat to medium-high and add the chopped bacon and shallots. Sauté for 2 minutes, then add the sliced mushrooms. Cook for a further 3 minutes, until the mushrooms soften, then stir in the garlic and thyme and cook for 1 minute. Pour in the stock and vinegar.

Add the chicken and bring to a simmer. Reduce the heat, cover and allow to simmer for 10 minutes until the chicken is cooked through (there should be no pink meat when you cut it open).

Stir in the spreadable cheese until it has melted into the sauce, and the sauce is smooth and creamy. Taste and add some freshly ground pepper to taste.

Remove from the heat and serve. The dish can be frozen once cooled – defrost thoroughly before reheating.

Day Six

BREAKFAST	VALUES
TOTAL	

LUNCH	VALUES
TOTAL	

DINNER	VALUES
TOTAL	

SNACKS AND TREATS	VALUES
TOTAL	

Notes

WATER

The BEST project

YOU'LL EVER WORK ON IS

YOU

Shopping List ②

....
....
....
....
....
....
....
....
....
....
....
....
....
....
....
....
....
....
....

Shopping List ①

....
....
....
....
....
....
....
....
....
....
....
....
....
....
....
....
....
....
....

Week **THIRTEEN** *done!*

BREAKFAST	VALUES
TOTAL	

LUNCH	VALUES
TOTAL	

DINNER	VALUES
TOTAL	

SNACKS AND TREATS	VALUES
TOTAL	

Notes

_____

_____

_____

WATER

◇ ◇ ◇ ◇
◇ ◇ ◇ ◇

Acknowledgements

Firstly we want to say a huge thank you to all of our followers on social media and all those who make our recipes. Without you, this planner and everything else we do just wouldn't be possible. Particular thanks to all who gave such amazing feedback on the first planner; you've helped shape this new, improved version!

Thank you to our publisher Carole, Martha, Bríd, Jodie and the rest of the team at Bluebird – you've been such an amazing part of the Pinch of Nom journey so far...!

Thanks to everyone at Nic & Lou, especially to Emma and Nikki. You guys always take what is in our heads and make it look 1000 times better.

To Becky for all your help navigating the tough stuff!

Special thanks go to Emma, Lisa and Meadows – thanks for all your hard work and your inspiration. Additional thanks go to Sophie, Katie, Matt, Stephen, Ellie, Lauren, Cheryl, Vince, Rubi and Sydney – thank you for making Nom work and for keeping everything ticking over. We're so proud to work with you lot.

Our thanks also to our amazing taste testing group for all your help in sending feedback and suggestions for these recipes. We have really appreciated the time you gave to support this project.

To our agent Clare, for believing in us from day one.

Thanks to Helen, Steve, Jen, Nick, Isla and Millie, and the rest of the Spence clan.

With thanks as ever to Paul – none of this would ever have been possible without your and Cath's support. This, alongside everything we do, will always be for Cath.

No acknowledgement would be complete without a mention for our various furry babies – Brandi, Ginger Cat and Freda.